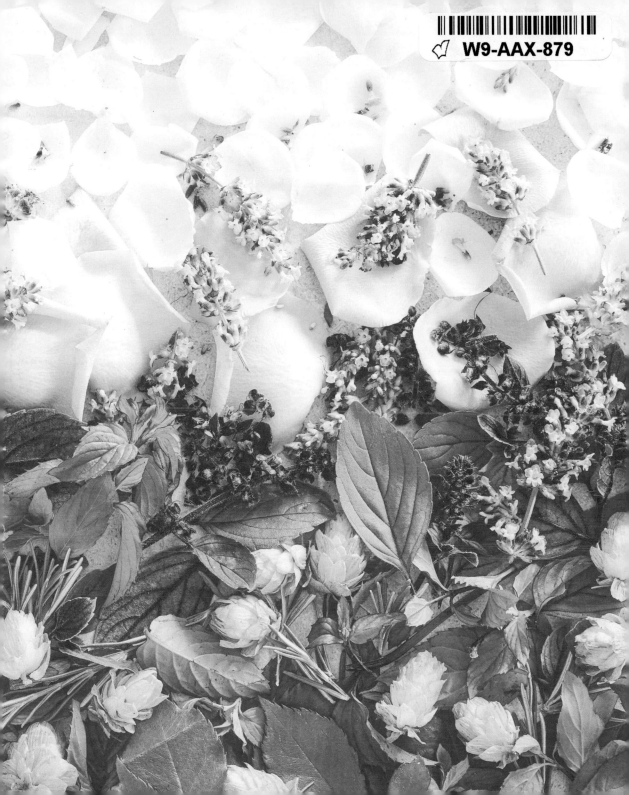

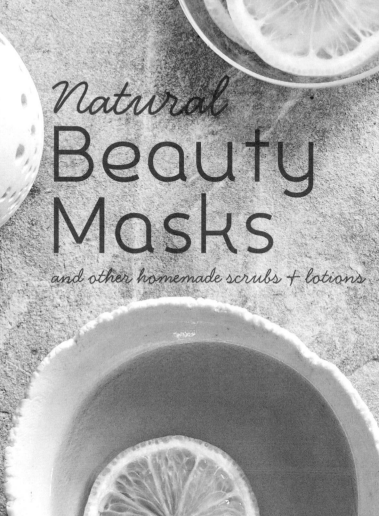

Natural
Beauty
Masks

and other homemade scrubs + lotions

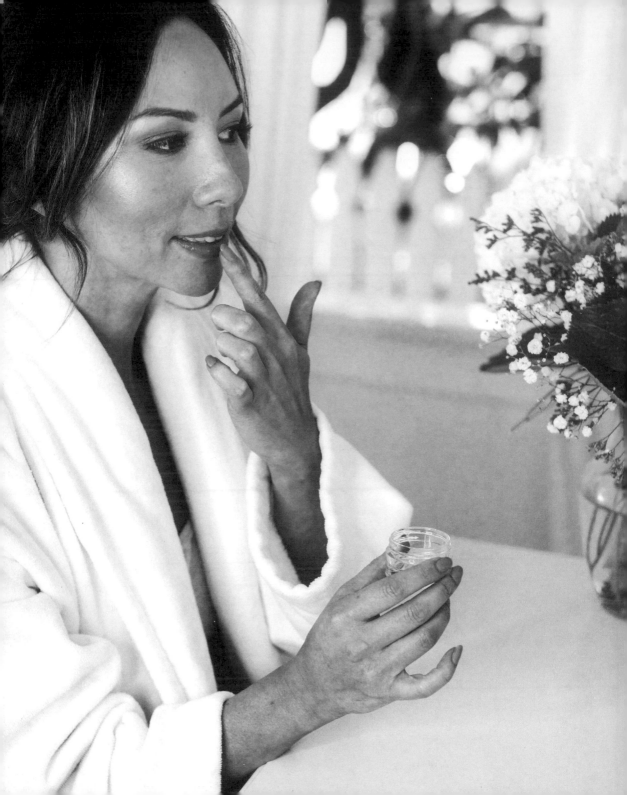

Natural Beauty Masks

and other homemade scrubs + lotions

Caroline Artiss

with photography by Mowie Kay

RYLAND PETERS & SMALL
LONDON • NEW YORK

Designer Barbara Zuñiga
Editor Miriam Catley
Production Controller Mai-Ling Collyer
Art director Leslie Harrington
Editorial director Julia Charles
Publisher Cindy Richards

Food stylists Kathy Kordalis and Sian Henley
Props stylist Olivia Wardle
Model photography by Samantha Klose
Still life photography by Mowie Kay

First published in 2018 by
Ryland Peters & Small
20–21 Jockey's Fields, London WC1R 4BW
and
341 E 116th St, New York NY 10029
www.rylandpeters.com

10 9 8 7 6 5 4 3 2 1

ISBN: 978-1-84975-942-7

Printed in China

A CIP record for this book is available from the British
Library. US Library of Congress Cataloging-in-
Publication Data has been applied for.

Disclaimer:
The views expressed in this book are those of the
author but they are general views only and readers
are urged to consult a relevant and qualified specialist
or physician for individual advice before beginning any
regimen. Ryland Peters & Small hereby exclude all
liability to the extent permitted by law for any errors
or omissions in this book and for any loss, damage or
expense (whether direct or indirect) suffered by a third
party relying on any information contained in this book.

*This book is dedicated to my late Mother,
Christina Pegg, Beautician, 1953–2015*

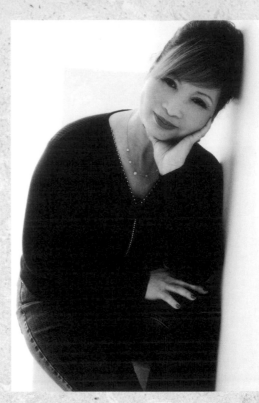

Notes:
· Both metric British (Metric) and American (Imperial
  plus US cups) measurements are included in these
  recipes for convenience; however it is important to
  work with one set of measurements and not
  alternate between the two within a recipe.
· Where possible choose organic ingredients.

Contents

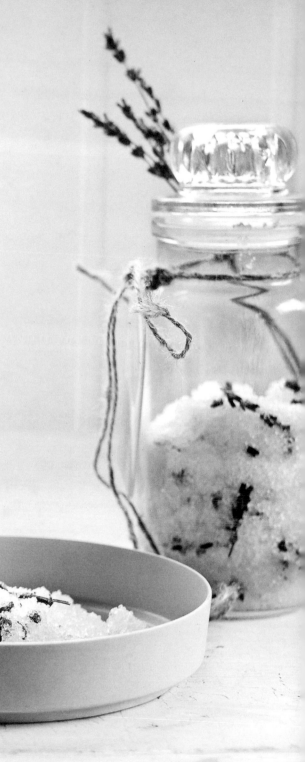

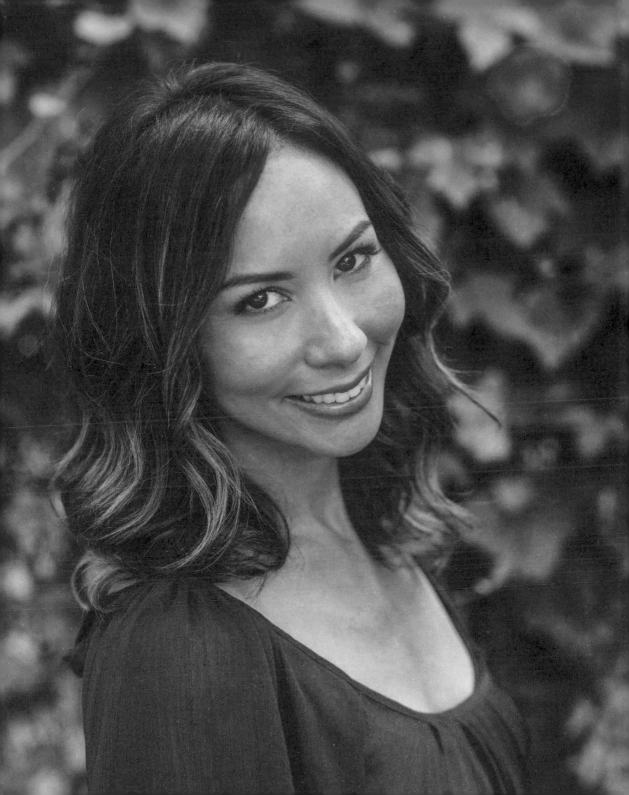

Introduction

I believe in an holistic approach to beauty. A healthy balanced diet full of fresh foods, drinking plenty of water to keep yourself hydrated and toxins flushed out, making sure you have enough sleep every night to help your body heal and restore itself, and using natural beauty treatments to help keep skin protected, cleansed and nourished from the outside are all important.

Food and natural ingredients have been used for centuries in beauty regimes and now most large cosmetic companies use elements derived from natural food sources to add nourishment to their skin care products. In my last book, I focused on creating specific recipes aimed at eating the right foods for all your beauty needs and to help you shine from the inside out. In this book, I have created recipes using natural ingredients that can be applied topically and will feed and nourish your skin from the outside. Not all ingredients that I used in my last book would be ideal to lather on your skin, I'm not sure I'd find it too relaxing laying down with a slice of raw salmon on my face! But there are plenty of natural foods that can be turned into face masks, such as avocados, bananas, strawberries, cucumbers, eggs, oats, yogurt and milk, to name a few. All these ingredients are easy to find and can do wonders for your skin.

My late mother was a well-established beautician and had her own beauty clinic, Hibiscus, in Stoke Poges, England. She taught me so much as I was growing up about how to take good care of my skin, and I want to share her advice with you. Every night before you go to sleep make sure you cleanse your face to wash off any excess dirt or oil, then use a toner to close and tighten the pores, and lastly moisturize to keep your skin soft. Exfoliate a couple of times a week, use a good face mask once every week or two, and always remember to apply a good SPF on your face to protect it from sun damage. It's simple but highly effective advice and I have my mother to thank for my healthy-looking skin. She studied aromatherapy, among many things, and used essential oils to help calm, heal and soothe. I like to add a drop or two to some of my masks for their natural benefits and their magical aromas. Certain aromas can evoke calming sensations, and can help the body heal naturally, and some essential oils can help awaken and invigorate the senses. She would always remind me to take great care when using essential oils for any beauty treatments as they are very potent and powerful, and always buy the purest quality you can find.

Ingredients Glossary

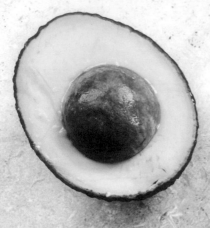

Activated charcoal draws out poisons, toxins and all the grease and dirt from your pores and surface of the skin.

Almond oil is derived from nutrient-rich almonds, which are high in unsaturated healthy fats and vitamins A and E. It is a mild, antioxidative and hypo-allergenic oil making it widely used in skin and hair treatments.

Aloe vera is a powerhouse of natural goodness. It has over 75 different vitamins, minerals, enzymes and natural compounds. It is widely used for healing and often used for soothing sunburnt skin.

Apple cider vinegar has many beauty benefits. It contains antiseptic, anti-fungal and anti-inflammatory properties. It is rich in acetic, malic and citric acids, which help soften the skin and remove residue build-ups. It also contains an abundance of vitamins, mineral salts, enzymes and amino acids.

Apricots contain essential fatty acids and vitamin A, making them perfect for feeding your skin and keeping it hydrated.

Avocados and avocado oil are a great source of healthy monounsaturated fats, vitamin B, potassium and vitamins A, C and E which are all essential for healthy skin.

Bananas are a rich source of potassium and contain vitamins E and C, all of which help promote clear glowing skin.

Beer contains hops, saccharides, yeast and B vitamins, all of which are great for skin and hair.

Bees wax forms a protective barrier for the skin, locking moisture in and protecting skin from toxins. It's a natural humectant, which draws in moisture. It's anti-allergenic and is used widely in lip balm.

Bentonite clay helps to remove and draw out toxins from the skin, and can help heal skin, reduce redness and inflammation. It also contains an abundance of natural minerals including calcium, magnesium, silica, sodium, copper, iron and potassium.

Bergamot essential oil helps soothe nerves and reduces tension, anxiety and stress, and provides skin purifying benefits.

Chamomile is known for its ability to help stomach aches and to promote feelings of calmness and relaxation. It also contains antioxidants and has anti-inflammatory properties.

Chia seeds are packed full of a wealth of nutrients. They contain a high amount of omega-3 fatty acids, which are essential to healthy glowing skin, plus calcium, magnesium, tryptophan, fibre and protein.

Cinnamon contains calcium, fibre, manganese and iron. It also has antiseptic and anti-microbial properties and it helps stimulate blood flow to the skin.

Cocoa is packed full of antioxidants that help repair damaged skin cells and neutralize free radicals. It contains over 300 compounds which are good for your health, including compounds that help boost endorphins and serotonin levels, which help make you feel happier.

Cocoa butter is a natural oil that comes from the cocoa bean. It's highly moisturizing and hydrating for your skin as it contains essential fatty acids. It is widely used in beauty products.

Coconut oil has many benefits for skin health including three different fatty acids that help retain moisture in the skin. It also contains strong disinfectant and antimicrobial properties, and vitamin E.

Coffee contains caffeine, which is used in many beauty treatments. It helps brighten skin and reduce inflammations. The coffee bean contains caffeic acid which can help boost collagen production. The grains make an excellent and gentle exfoliator.

Coffee berry is the fruit surrounding the coffee bean. It's called a superfood due the exceptionally high levels of antioxidants, vitamins, minerals and plant polyphenols. These help fight free radicals that lead to skin damage. Coffee berries also contain immune-boosting, anti-inflammatory and anti-viral properties.

Cucumber is full of soothing and astringent properties and they help revitalize skin. They are 96 per cent water, which helps hydrate dry skin, and they contain potassium, magnesium, biotin, vitamins A, B1 and C.

Eggs are a rich source of fats and proteins that aid in moisturizing your skin, help tighten skin and reduce pores.

Epsom salts are a mineral compound of magnesium and sulphate. These are both essential minerals for our bodies. Soaking in Epsom salts can help relieve aching muscles and dry skin.

Eucalyptus oil has many medicinal properties, such as being anti-inflammatory, anti-spasmodic, a decongestant, antibacterial and antiseptic. It can be used to help alleviate aching muscles.

Gelatine is a source of animal protein. It contains collagen and essential amino acids, such as lysine, proline and glycine. These help repair connective tissue and regulate cell function, which helps with firmer, tighter, more youthful skin.

Ginger has over 40 antioxidant properties and is antiseptic in nature. It can help increase blood circulation and has been used for centuries in ancient healing medicines. The antioxidants help protect the skin cells from damage.

Grapefruit essential oil contains large amounts of the photochemical bromelain, which is a complex mix of enzymes that have an anti inflammatory effect, help boost fat cell metabolism and can help to reduce cellulite.

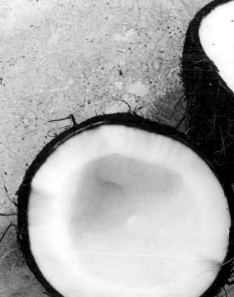

Honey, raw honey in particular, contains many natural healing properties, it's a natural moisturizer, contains vitamins and minerals plus antioxidants, it's a humectant and it has antimicrobial properties.

Jojoba oil is used widely in beauty treatments. It is rich in essential nutrients, such as iodine, and antioxidants, vitamins E and B complex, silicon, zinc and copper. It is similar to the natural sebum our skin produces and it helps to moisturize and keep our oil levels balanced without clogging our pores.

Lavender essential oil helps reduce stress and anxiety. It's known to aid healing of wounds, alleviate headaches, help with sleep, and contains antioxidants that are good for the skin.

Lemons are rich in vitamin C, which is an antioxidant that helps protect the skin against cell damage. It is also antibacterial and contains citric acid which helps with acne, blemishes and oily skin.

Lemon essential oil is widely used for its stimulating yet calming properties. It enhances mood and concentration. It's antiseptic, an astringent, anti-fungal and detoxifying.

Lemongrass is a natural astringent, naturally antiseptic, and anti fungal and works as a great cleanser for skin.

Mayonnaise is made of eggs and oil which make it a natural skin and hair hydrator that will help preserve moisture.

Milk has been used in beauty regimes for centuries. It contains beneficial nutrients, such as calcium, lactic acid, vitamins A, D, B6 and B12, selenium, potassium, biotin and protein.

Natural yogurt is great for your skin as it contains lactic acid, which can help get rid of dead skin, clear blemishes, tighten pores and can help with skin discolouration. It also contains calcium, zinc and B vitamins.

Oats contain 18 different amino acids, which are essential for rebuilding and repairing skin tissue. It's also a humectant, which means it helps your skin retain moisture. It's hypo-allergenic and works well as an exfoliant.

Olive oil is a great natural moisturizer and contains three major antioxidants, Vitamin E, which is widely used in skin care products, plus polyphenols and phytosterols. These antioxidants help to fight free radicals, which can cause skin damage and early skins of aging.

Papaya is a tropical fruit rich in vitamins A, C, E and K, magnesium, potassium, niacin, carotene, protein, fibre, and the enzyme papain, which helps cleanse the skin. The fruit is antioxidant-rich, which helps protect skin, while brightening and getting rid of clogged pores.

Peaches are a great source of vitamins A and C, and selenium. Vitamins A and C help protect and regenerate skin tissue.

Peppermint essential oil has antibacterial properties and has been used to relieve bad breath and some digestive problems. It also has a cooling and soothing effect and can be used on aching muscles.

Potatoes are rich in minerals, sulphur, phosphorous and potassium. Potato juice contains vitamin C and antioxidant properties, which can improve skin tone, lighten skin, and help with dark circles under the eyes. They also contain anti-inflammatory and astringent properties which can help relieve puffy eyes.

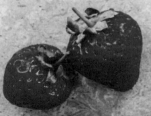

Raspberries are rich in vitamins, antioxidants, phytonutrients, anthocyanins and fibre and also a high concentration of ellagic acid. They help protect the skin from harmful free radicals that break down skin cells.

Rose essential oil has been known to help improve depression, relieve anxiety, help with problem skin conditions like acne, and increase libido.

Rosewater is a great natural skin cleanser as it contains anti-inflammatory properties, which can help reduce redness and soothe skin.

Rosemary essential oil is packed full of antioxidants, antibacterial and anti-inflammatory properties, plus it acts as a stimulant.

Sea salt is a natural detoxifier and it helps absorb toxins from your skin when you bath in it, and it helps your skin retain its moisture. Sea salt contains essential natural minerals that our skin and bodies need, such as magnesium, calcium, potassium and sodium.

Shea butter helps repair skin and boost collagen. It contains great amounts of vitamins A and E, and is rich in oleic and stearic acids. It is a highly moisturizing and hydrating skin agent. It can help reduce inflammation and has anti-aging properties.

Spirulina is a superfood made from green algae. It contains a large amount of protein, vitamins A, K1, K2 and B12, iron, manganese, chromium and phytonutrients.

Strawberries contain a large amount of vitamin C which is a natural antioxidant that helps fight free radicals, which can damage skin cells and break down collagen.

Sugar, both white and brown sugars, are a natural humectant, which means they help draw moisture into the skin keeping it hydrated. Sugar is also a natural source of glycolic acid, an alpha hydroxy acid, which encourages cell turnover for fresher, younger-looking skin. The fine particles of the sugar act as an exfoliant.

Sweet orange essential oil is used widely as a mood enhancer and is known to have many uplifting and anti depressant properties.

Tea tree oil contains powerful antiseptic, anti-fungal and anti-inflammatory properties. It has been used to treat skin conditions such as acne, psoriasis, eczema, nail fungus and more.

Tomatoes are rich in lycopene, a powerful antioxidant and an astringent, which helps tighten pores. They contain natural acids that help regulate oily skin.

Turmeric is high in antioxidants, which help prevent skin cell damage. It also contains anti-inflammatory properties that can help with skin conditions such as acne, dry skin, psoriasis and eczema. Turmeric is also known to help brighten skin.

Vanilla contains many antioxidants including vanillic acid and vanillin. These help protect the skin from harmful free radicals and toxins.

Vitamin E oil is a fat-soluble antioxidant and nutrient for your skin. It helps fight free radicals that can damage skin cells. It helps support new skin cell growth and regeneration, while boosting collagen production.

Tips for your home spa

Do a patch test Everyone's skin reacts differently to creams and ingredients, so the best way to make sure you find the perfect face masks and treatments for your skin is to do a small patch test on your skin first. Dab a little of the new face mask onto the skin underneath your forearm as the skin is thinner. Keep it on for 10 minutes. If you feel any bad reaction like redness, itching or soreness, then it means your skin isn't agreeing with the raw ingredients.

Face mask essentials Always apply face masks to clean, make-up-free skin. Wash the face mask off using your hands or a clean face cloth with warm water, and continue with your regular daily face cleansing routine.

Natural cleaning tips Body scrubs that contain ingredients such as coffee grains can leave the bath tub looking a bit of a fright, and most of my body scrubs contain natural oils, which can leave a slippery surface. A great natural cleaning solution I make at home is a simple solution of white vinegar and water mixed to the ratio of 50/50. Keep it in a spray bottle and squirt on areas to get rid of grease and dirt. Wherever possible choose natural cleaning products for your home.

Use dark or old towels Ingredients such as turmeric, charcoal and spirulina have such a deep colour that they can stain.

Useful equipment Luckily to make DIY beauty masks at home you don't need any special equipment, just a bowl and a spoon and fork mainly to mix and mash things up in. I have a **small blender** at home that I use to finely blend some of my masks. A hand-held stick blender or a small food processor would do just as good a job, and if you don't have either then a fork will do but it just takes a bit longer.

I find it very handy to have a stock of **small jars with lids** for keeping some of the body scrubs and lip treatments in as some of them last for several weeks. If you are feeling in a generous mood they also make wonderful homemade gifts.

I like to apply my face masks with a **large, flat make-up brush,** or you can buy special brushes for applying face masks too, just like the ones they use in the beauty spas.

I recommend treating yourself to a special **foot bath,** one you can keep in the cupboard for the times your feet need a relaxing soak at the end of the day. There are so many available to choose from, and some even have air streams for bubbles and massagers to take the aches and pains away.

Other items that are handy to have around are a **shower cap** if you're doing a hair mask, **hair clips and ties,** a **body brush** for exfoliating, and a **pumice stone** or some kind of foot exfoliator for the tougher skin areas.

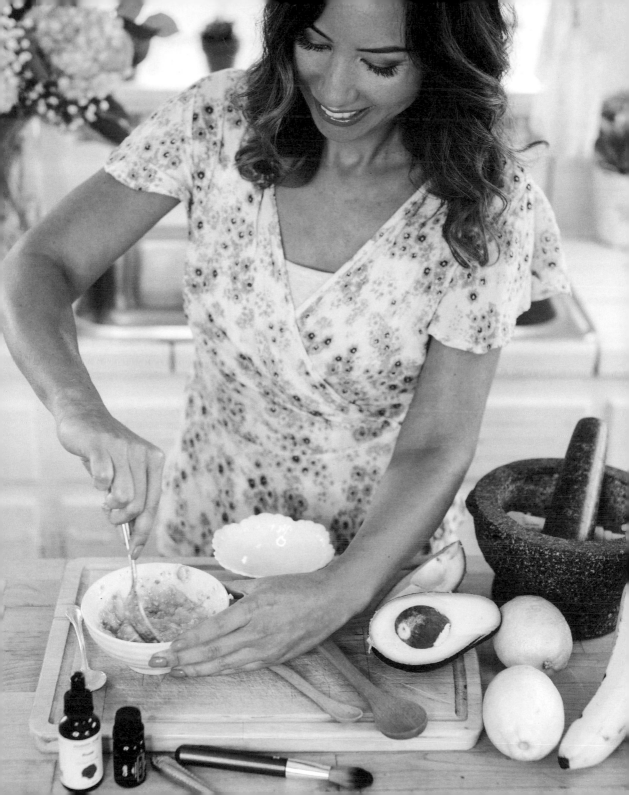

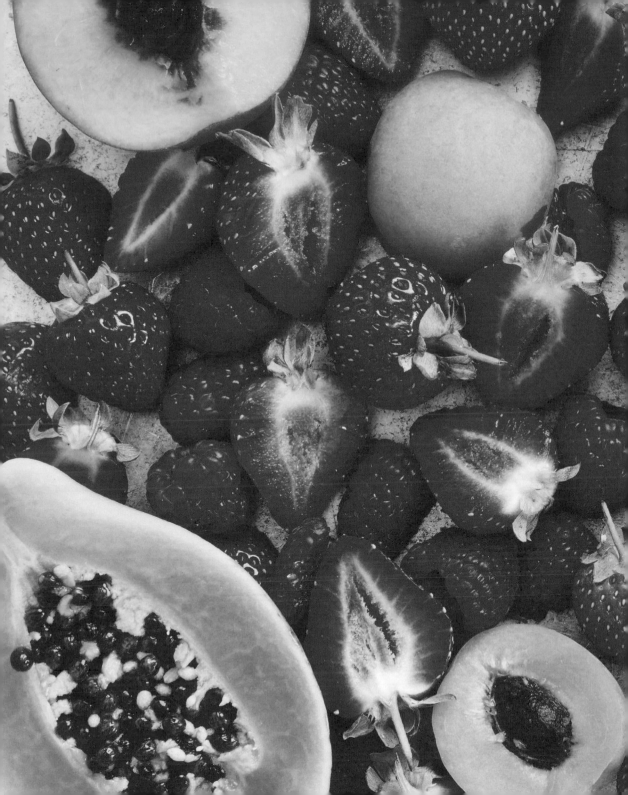

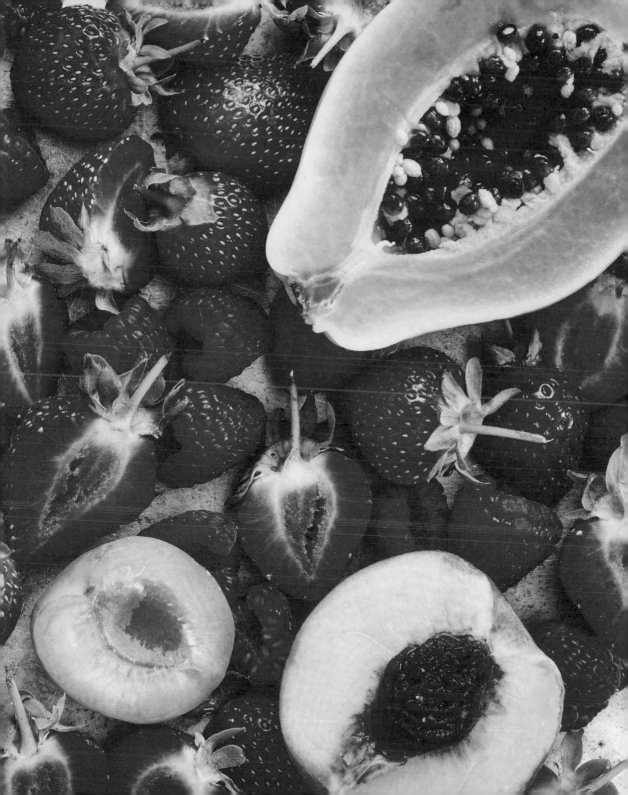

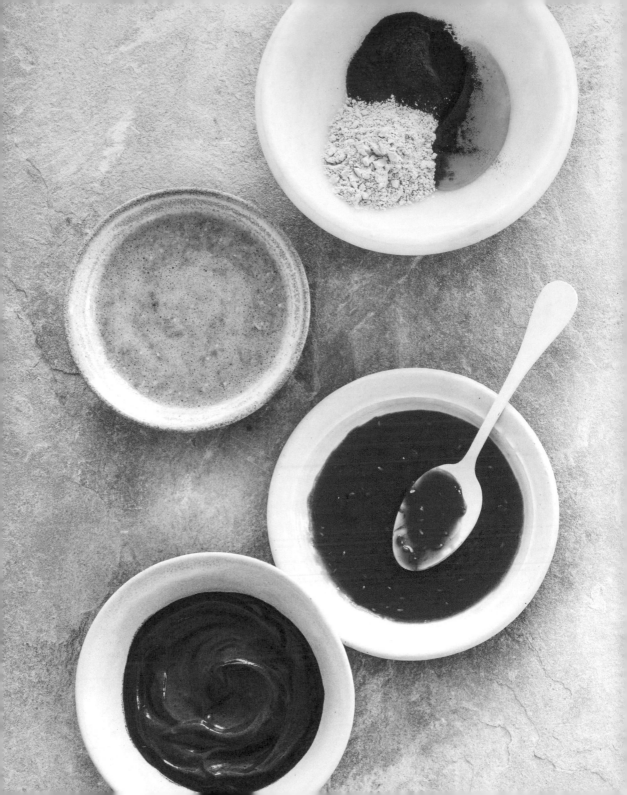

face masks
+ exfoliators

Face masks can be used to detoxify, cleanse, hydrate, moisturize
and nourish your skin. They can also help remove excess oil
from your face and tighten pores. We all have different skin types
and requirements so I have created face masks for oily skin,
combination skin, dry skin and normal skin. Each face mask
recipe yields just enough for one or two applications and some
can be kept in the refrigerator to treat yourself another day.
As the ingredients in the masks are fresh, they won't keep for as
long as shop-bought beauty products, but the advantage is you
are feeding your skin with the vitamins and minerals it needs
straight from the source without any chemical preservatives,
not to mention saving a whole bunch of money.

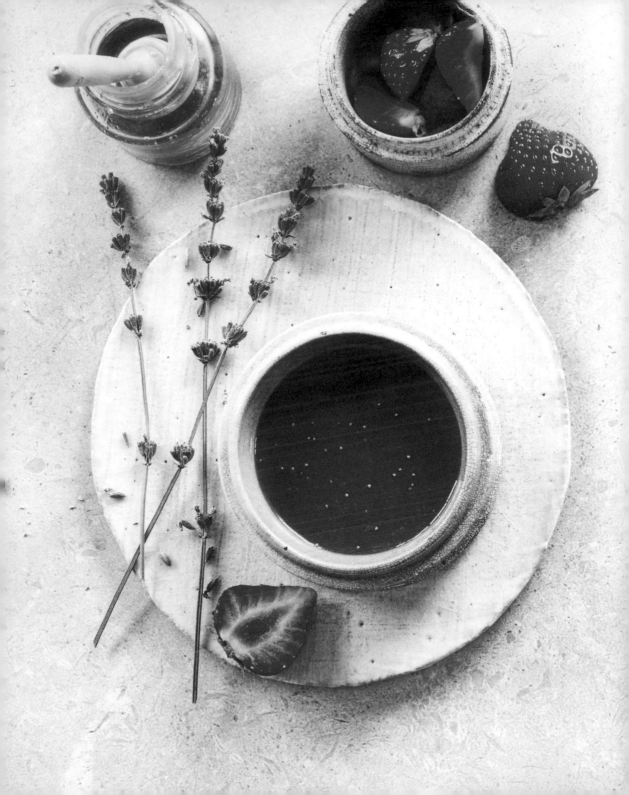

Strawberry + Lavender Face Mask

for normal/combination skin

Strawberries contain alpha hydroxy acids, and lots of vitamin C, which helps to feed and protect the skin and works as an exfoliant, too. Honey is fantastic for the skin because it is a natural moisturizer and is packed full of antimicrobial, antioxidant and humectant properties.

50 g/ ½ cup (or 3 medium-large) strawberries,
*   washed and hulled*
1 tablespoon raw organic honey
1 teaspoon avocado oil
1 drop lavender essential oil

Makes 2–3 applications
Keeps for 3 days in the refrigerator

Put all the ingredients in a small food processor and pulse until you have a fine purée.

Use a large face-mask brush to spread the mixture evenly over your clean face, avoiding the eye area. Leave it on for 10–15 minutes, then wash it off with warm water and gently pat the skin dry.

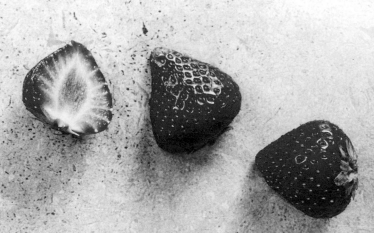

Spirulina + Yogurt Face Mask

for normal skin

Commonly found at health food stores, spirulina is a powerhouse of nutrients with antibacterial properties, which helps to both nourish the skin and keep pores clean and tight, thus preventing outbreaks of spots or blemishes. Yogurt helps to soothe and purify the skin, while olive oil adds a natural moisturizing effect and is loaded with antioxidants, which help to reduce fine lines and fight the free radicals caused by exposure to the sun's UV rays.

2 tablespoons natural full-fat Greek yogurt
1 teaspoon extra virgin olive oil
1 teaspoon spirulina powder

Makes 2–3 applications
Keeps for up to 3 days in the refrigerator

Mix all the ingredients together in a small bowl.

Using a large face-mask brush, clean fingers or the back of a spoon, spread the mixture over your clean face, avoiding the eye area. Leave it on for 10–15 minutes, then wash it off with warm water and gently pat the skin dry.

Note: This mask will stain, so be careful not to let it come into contact with any white or precious clothes.

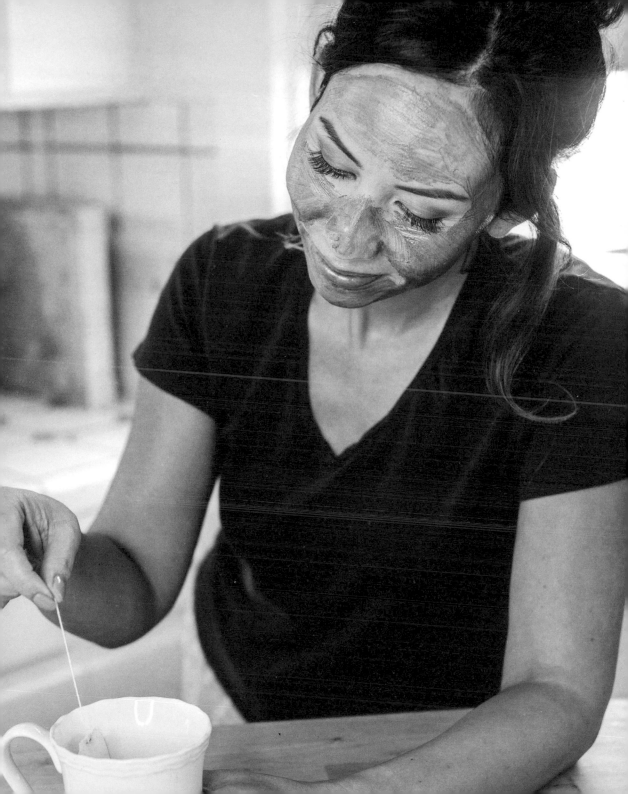

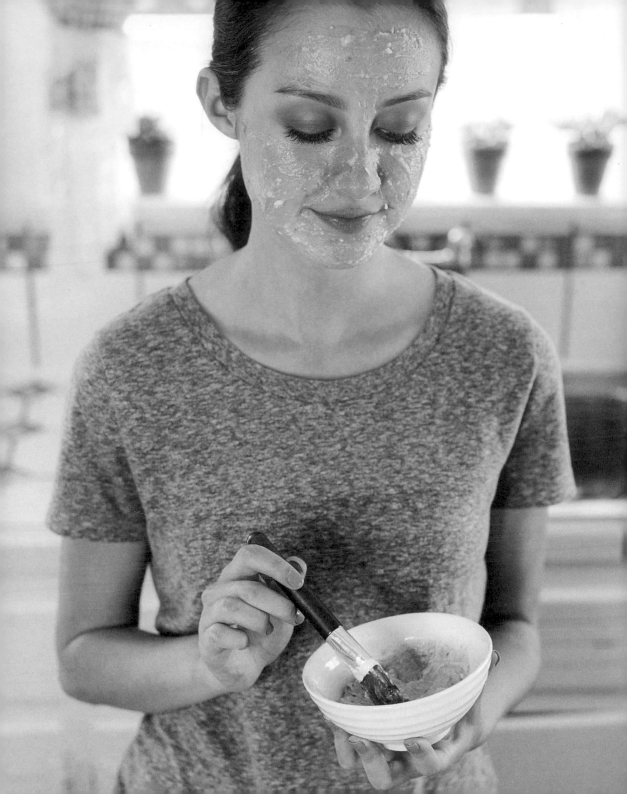

Avocado + Banana Face Mask

for normal to dry skin

Avocados are fantastic fruits for their skin benefits. They are a rich source of vitamins A, C and E, all of which are essential for healthy, glowing skin. Vitamin E is also an antioxidant that helps to repair and protect the skin. Bananas are a rich source of potassium and have been used in home skin care remedies for centuries, to keep skin moisturized and plump.

¼ ripe avocado (flesh only)
¼ ripe banana, peeled
1 tablespoon raw organic honey
1 teaspoon avocado oil

Makes 2 applications
Keeps for up to 1 day in the refrigerator

Put all the ingredients in a small food processor and pulse until you have a fine purée; alternatively, you can mash them together in a bowl using a fork.

Using a large face-mask brush or clean fingers, spread the mixture over your clean face, avoiding the eye area. Leave it on for 10–15 minutes, then wash it off with warm water and gently pat the skin dry.

Note: If an avocado has turned a bit too brown to eat, then this is the perfect time to mash it up and use it for a face mask.

Recipe idea: Banana + Avocado Smoothie

Using nearly all the same ingredients as the face mask, you can make yourself a delicious and healthy smoothie. In Vietnam, a popular smoothie is made out of just-ripe avocados and milk. It's one of my favourites, and the addition of the banana gives it some natural sweetness. Try this recipe when you make the face mask.

¼ ripe avocado (flesh only)
½ ripe banana, peeled
1 tablespoon raw organic honey
240 ml/1 cup milk (almond, coconut or cow's milk)

Serves 1

Blend all the ingredients together in a blender with 2–3 ice cubes, pour into a glass and serve.

Lemon + Turmeric Face Mask

for oily-prone skin

This face mask leaves the skin feeling clean, less greasy and firmer than before. The citric acid content of the lemon juice helps to tighten and minimize pores, while turmeric is a great anti-inflammatory and helps to reduce dark spots and blemishes. I like to use freshly grated turmeric root because it contains more active ingredients than the powder, but you can use turmeric powder if you can't get hold of the fresh root.

1 egg white
1 teaspoon freshly squeezed lemon juice
2 tablespoons ground rolled oats or oatmeal
½ teaspoon freshly grated turmeric root or turmeric powder

Makes enough for 1 application
Keeps for up to 1 day in the refrigerator

Put the egg white in a bowl and beat with a fork or whisk until frothy. Add the lemon juice, oats or oatmeal and turmeric and whisk together.

Using a large face-mask brush or clean fingers, apply the face mask to freshly cleaned skin, avoiding the eye area. Lie down with an old towel under your head and relax for 10 minutes, then wash it off with cool to warm water and gently pat the skin dry.

Notes: It's advisable that you don't wear your best clothes or use white facecloths or towels when using this mask because turmeric will stain – although luckily it doesn't stain the skin. The oats give this mask a thicker consistency so it shouldn't run off your face when you apply it.

I like to grind up a couple of cups of rolled oats at one time and keep them in an airtight container for future use.

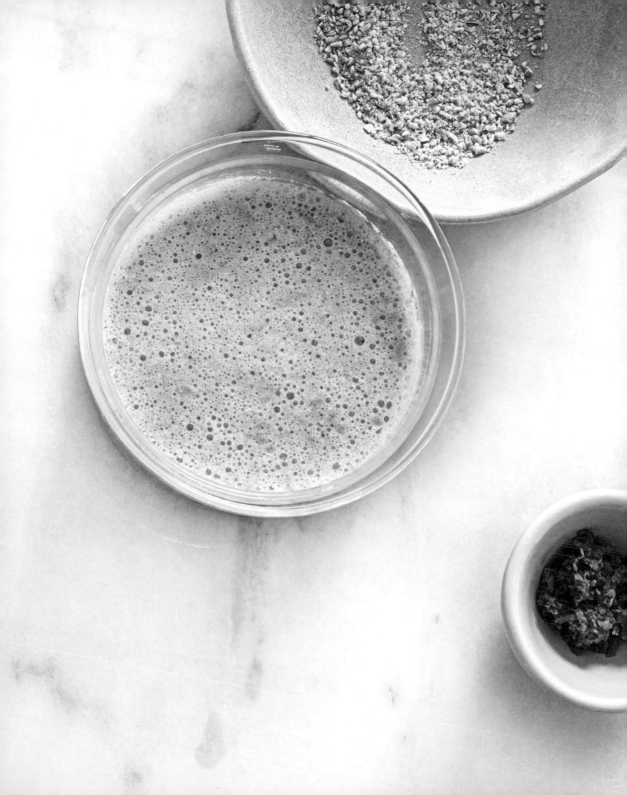

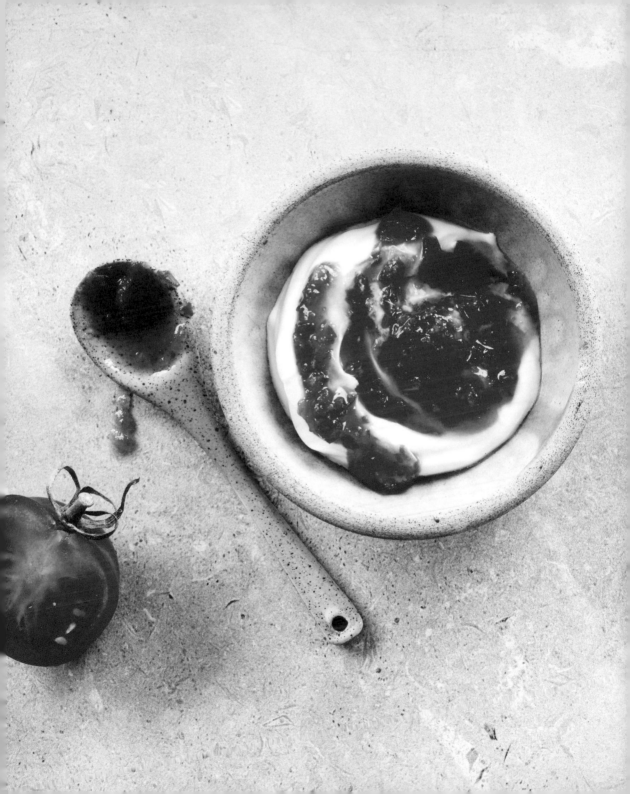

Tomato, Honey + Yogurt Face Mask

for oily-prone skin

Tomatoes have clarifying and astringent properties that help to absorb excess oil from the skin, while honey has antibacterial properties, and yogurt helps to bind it all together into a soothing face mask.

½ ripe medium-sized tomato
1 tablespoon raw organic honey
1 tablespoon natural full-fat Greek yogurt

Makes 2–3 applications
Keeps for up to 2 days in the refrigerator

Scoop the seeds out of the tomato and discard. Put the tomato and honey into a small food processor and whizz them together until smooth. Put the yogurt in a small bowl and stir in the tomato mixture.

This mask can be a bit runny, so use a large face-mask brush to apply a layer to freshly cleaned skin, avoiding the eye area. Leave it on for 10 minutes, then wash it off with warm water and gently pat the skin dry.

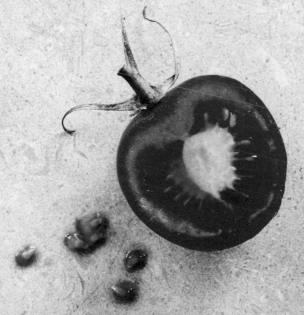

Cooling Cucumber, Tea Tree + Mint Face Mask

for oily-prone skin

Cucumbers are packed full of soothing and astringent properties, which is why they are often used in eye treatments and face masks. The oatmeal helps to remove dead skin cells and unblock pores, leaving skin clearer. Tea tree oil is a natural astringent and so helps to reduce excess oil on the skin, tighten the pores and fight acne.

¼ small cucumber
2 fresh mint leaves, or 2 drops peppermint essential oil
25 g / ¼ cup ground rolled oats
1½ tablespoons natural low-fat Greek yogurt
1 drop tea tree essential oil

Makes 2 applications
Keeps for up to 2 days in the refrigerator

Using a small food processor, whizz everything together until you have a smooth, thick paste.

Using a large face-mask brush or clean fingers, apply the mask to freshly cleaned skin, avoiding the eye area, and leave it on for 10 minutes. Wash it off with warm water and pat the skin dry.

Recipe idea: Cucumber + Mint Refresher

Try adding a few slices of cucumber and a few torn or bruised mint leaves to a glass of still or sparkling water. They add a wonderfully refreshing taste that will encourage you to drink more water. Ensuring you are well hydrated makes the skin look plumper and helps to flush toxins out of the body, which in turn keeps the skin clearer.

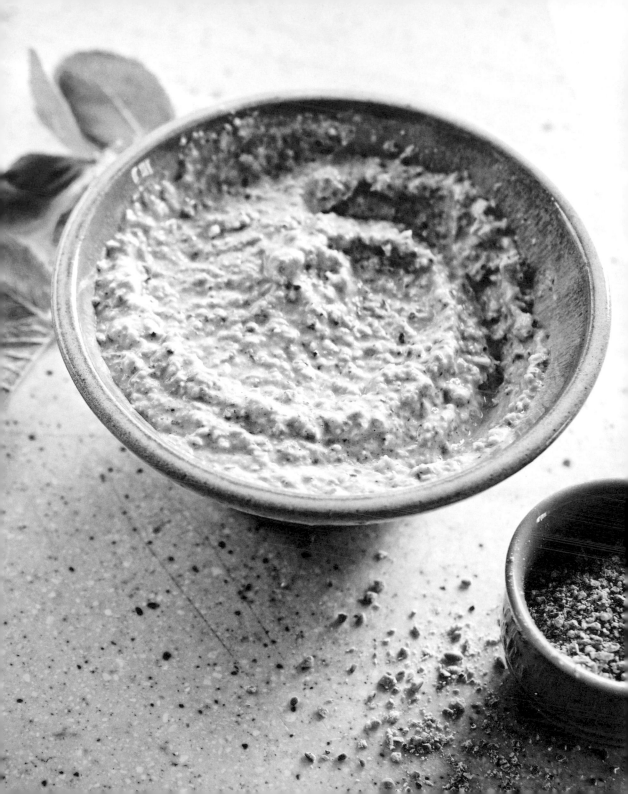

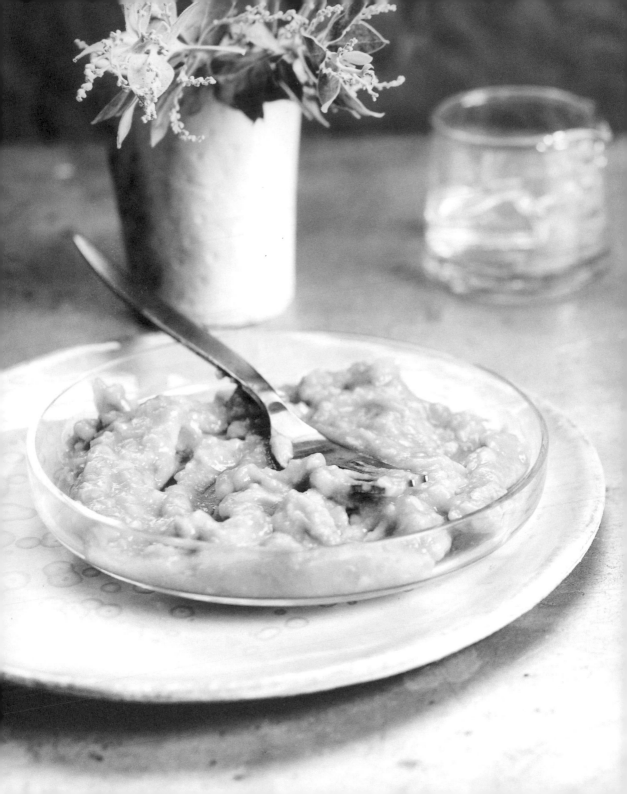

Avocado, Coconut Oil + Aloe Vera Face Mask

for dry skin

This face mask is made from a combination of three highly moisturizing beauty ingredients, resulting in a super-hydrating treatment for dry and flaky skin. Avocados are not only good for your skin when you eat them, but they are also fantastic to apply topically to hydrate, moisturize and pump your face full of skin-loving vitamin E and antioxidants. Coconut oil is an excellent natural moisturizer and has antibacterial and antimicrobial properties that help to keep skin clear. Aloe vera also has a wealth of natural skin benefits.

¼ ripe avocado (flesh only)
1 teaspoon pure organic coconut oil
1 tablespoon pure aloe vera gel

Makes 1 application
Keeps for up to 1 day in the refrigerator

You can make this face mask by hand or by using a small food processor. Scoop the avocado into a bowl and mash with a fork until it's smooth. Stir in the coconut oil, then add the aloe vera gel.

Using a large face-mask brush or clean fingers, apply the mask to your clean face, avoiding the eye area, and sit back and relax for 10–15 minutes. Wash it off with warm water and gently pat the skin dry.

Banana, Honey + Cinnamon Face Mask

for dry skin

Using fresh, ripe bananas on your face helps to brighten and moisturize dull, dry skin. Honey has excellent healing properties and acts as a humectant, which simply means it helps to retain and lock in moisture, keeping the skin well hydrated. Cinnamon helps to prevent acne because it is packed full of antibacterial and anti-fungal properties. It also stimulates blood flow to the skin, keeping it plump, and acts as a gentle exfoliant.

¼ ripe banana, peeled
½ tablespoon raw organic honey
½ teaspoon ground cinnamon
1 tablespoon ground rolled oats

Makes 2 applications

Keeps for up to 1 day in the refrigerator

Mash all the ingredients together in a small bowl until smooth, or use a small food processor.

Using a large face-mask brush or clean fingers, apply the mask to clean skin, avoiding the eye area. Leave it on for 10–15 minutes, then wash it off with warm water and gently pat the skin dry.

Recipe idea: Banana Toast

For a quick, healthy snack, top a piece of wholemeal/wholewheat toast with a few slices of banana, a drizzle of honey and a sprinkle of ground cinnamon. Put it under the grill/broiler set to a medium heat until the honey and banana start to caramelize. Serve.

Serves 1

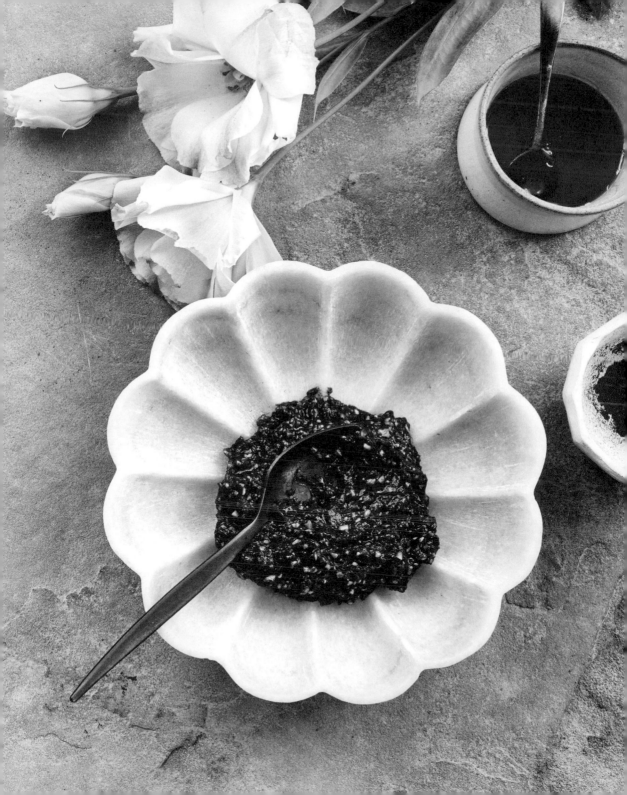

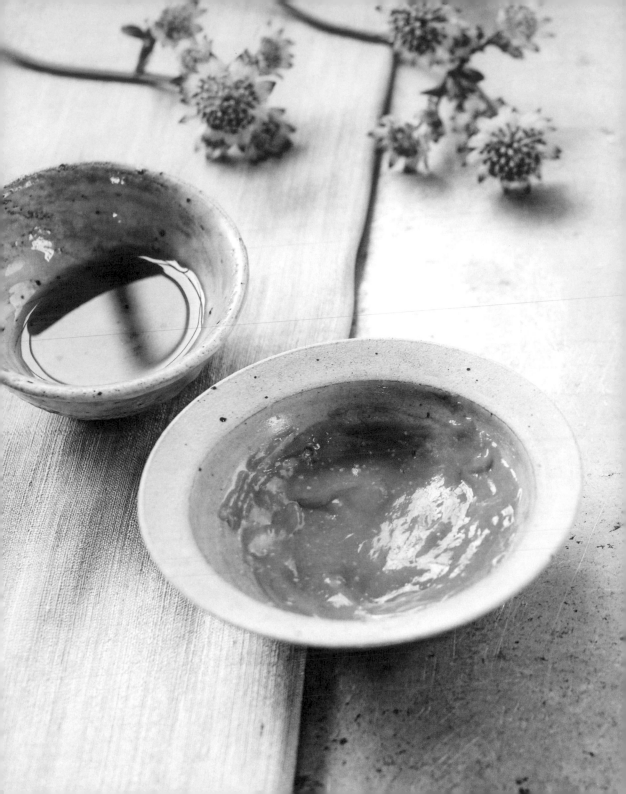

Olive Oil + Milk Face Mask

for dry skin

Olive oil is a great natural skin moisturizer and milk helps to soothe dry skin; I prefer to use an organic milk powder for face masks because it makes a paste that is ideal for spreading on the skin. Egg yolk is packed full of good fats that help to hydrate and add moisture back into the skin.

2 teaspoons extra virgin olive oil
1 tablespoon organic full-fat milk powder
1 egg yolk

Makes 2 applications
Keeps for up to 1–2 days in the refrigerator

Put all the ingredients into a small bowl and mix until you have a smooth, thick paste.

This mask has a beautiful, butter-like consistency, so you can use your fingers to smooth it over clean skin, avoiding the eye area. Leave it on for 10–15 minutes, before washing it off with cool to warm water and gently patting dry, for soft, glowing skin.

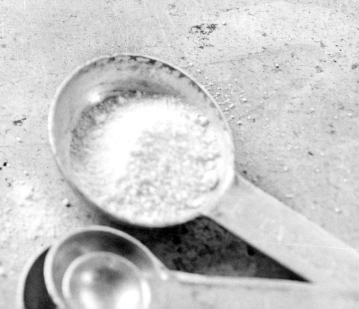

Papaya + Chia Seed Face Mask

for combination/normal skin

Rich in skin-friendly omega-3 essential fatty acids, chia seeds help to keep the skin hydrated, reduce inflammation and dryness, and increase circulation. Fresh papaya is great for all skin types as it is packed full of betacarotene, vitamin A and minerals to feed the skin. Honey has antibacterial properties to cleanse the skin while also adding moisture, and egg white has a firming, pore-tightening effect.

1 tablespoon ripe papaya flesh
1 egg white
1½ teaspoons raw organic honey
1½ teaspoons chia seeds

Makes 1–2 applications
Keeps for up to 1 day, covered, in the refrigerator

Scoop the papaya into a bowl and mash it with a fork until smooth. In a separate bowl, beat the egg white until frothy. Add 1 tablespoon of the egg white to the mashed papaya, along with the honey and chia seeds. Stir the ingredients together and leave in the refrigerator for 10 minutes. The chia seeds will give the mask a consistency similar to jelly/Jell-O and then it is ready to apply.

Using a large face-mask brush or clean fingers, spread the mixture evenly over clean skin, avoiding the eye area. Leave it on for 15 minutes, then wash it off with warm water and gently pat the skin dry.

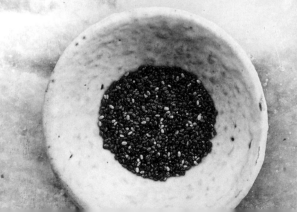

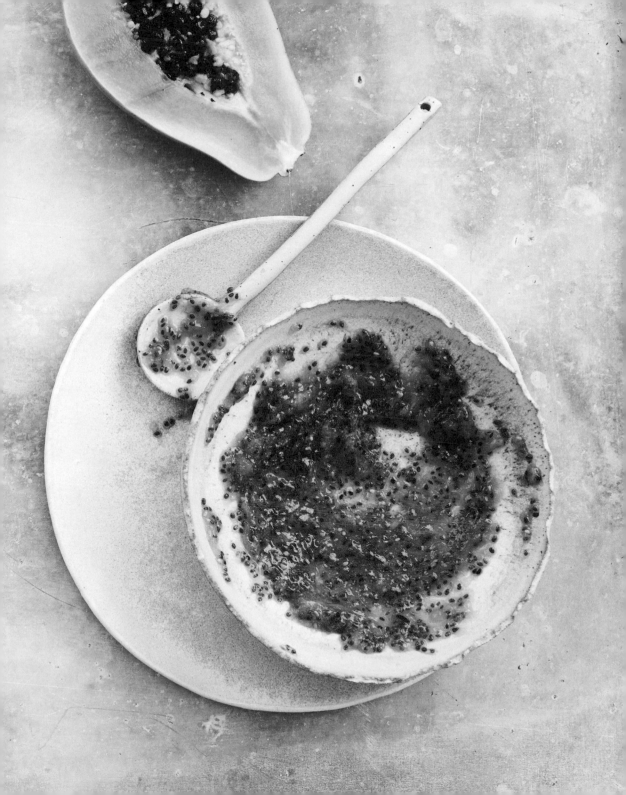

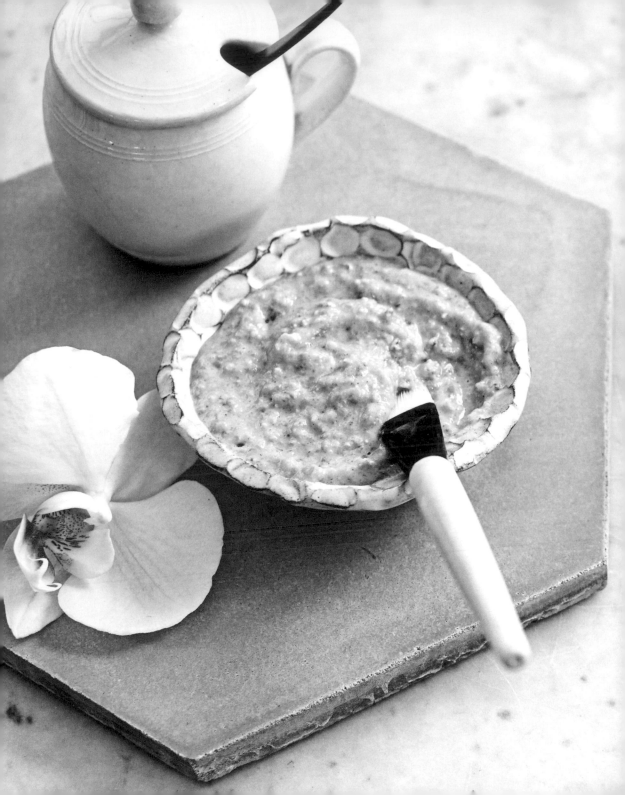

Apricot + Honey Face Mask

for combination/normal skin

The perfect blend of beauty-enhancing ingredients that work their magic on normal or combination skin, this face mask includes apricots, which are rich in vitamin A and a wonderful addition for promoting smoother, softer skin. It's literally good enough to eat (see below).

4 dried apricots
60 ml/¼ cup warm full-fat milk
25 g/¼ cup ground rolled oats
1 tablespoon raw organic honey

Makes 2 applications
Keeps for up to 2 days in the refrigerator

Simply put all the ingredients into a small food processor and whizz until you have a smooth paste.

Using a large face-mask brush or clean fingers, apply the paste generously to clean skin, avoiding the eye area. Leave it on for 15 minutes, then wash it off with warm water and gently pat the skin dry.

Recipe idea: Apricot and Honey Oatmeal

When I first made this face mask at home I just couldn't help but taste it. I was pleasantly surprised, so I decided to turn this face mask recipe into breakfast the next day.

50 g/½ cup ground rolled oats
5–6 dried apricots, chopped
250 ml/1 cup milk (almond, coconut or cow's milk)
1 tablespoon toasted flaked/slivered almonds
1–2 teaspoons raw organic honey
Serves 1

Put the oats, half of the chopped apricots and the milk into a small saucepan. Cook over a low heat, stirring continuously, until the oats have turned into thick oatmeal. Add more milk if you prefer a runnier consistency. Pour into a bowl and sprinkle the remaining apricots and the toasted almonds on top, then drizzle with honey to serve.

Charcoal Face Mask

for detoxifying

Activated charcoal is a natural, powerful, deep-cleansing ingredient, which works by drawing out toxins, chemicals and dirt from the skin, leaving the pores cleaner and less visible. It makes a great addition to your beauty cupboard at home, to help you achieve flawless skin.

1 teaspoon activated charcoal powder
1 teaspoon apple cider vinegar
1 drop tea tree essential oil
1 tablespoon natural full-fat Greek yogurt

Makes 1 application
Use same day

Put all the ingredients in a small bowl and stir together.

Using a face-mask brush, apply the mixture to clean skin, avoiding the delicate eye area. Leave it on for 10–15 minutes, then wash it off with warm water and gently pat the skin dry.

Note: Charcoal stains, so be careful not to let the face mask come into contact with white towels or clothes.

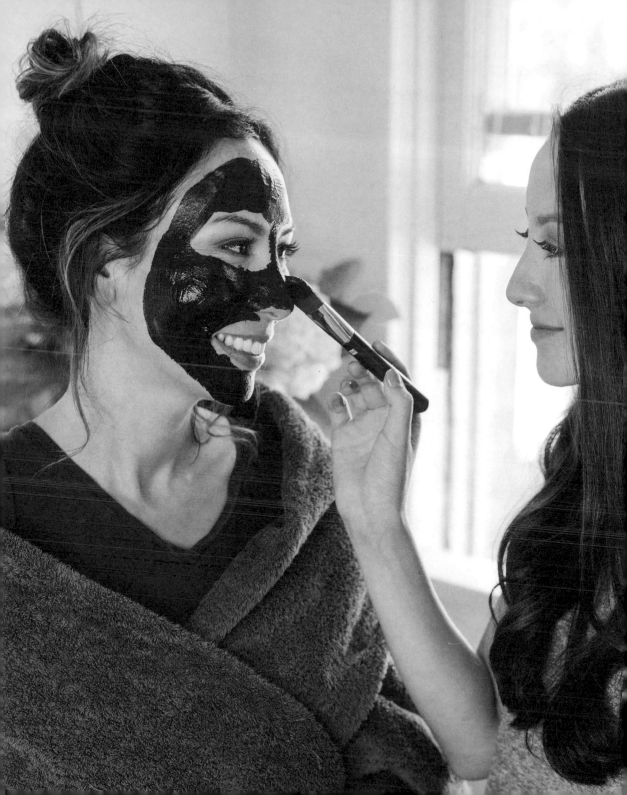

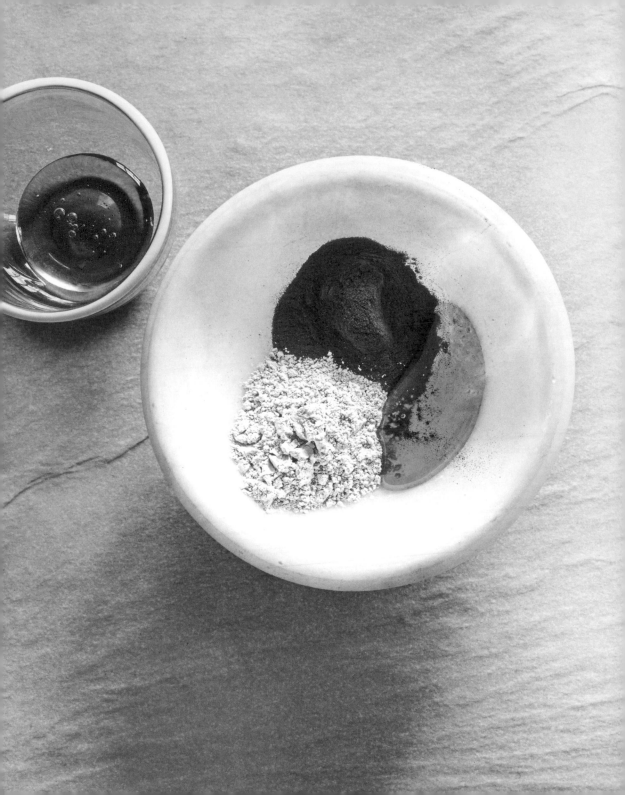

Bentonite Clay Detoxifying Face Mask

for detoxifying

There is so much we can learn about natural beauty from ancient remedies. Bentonite clay has been used for centuries in beauty and health regimes, and is a known beauty secret of the ancient Aztecs. It contains many skin-nourishing nutrients, such as iron, magnesium, calcium and sodium. When used as a beauty treatment on the skin it acts as an absorptive, which means it draws dirt, toxins, oil and grease out of the pores. The accumulation of dirt in the skin's pores leads to blackheads and larger, more visible pores.

1 tablespoon bentonite clay powder
1 teaspoon spirulina or kelp powder
1 teaspoon raw organic honey
1 tablespoon purified water

Makes 1 application
Use same day

Put all the ingredients in a small bowl and stir together.

Using a face-mask brush, apply the mixture to clean, dry skin, avoiding the delicate eye area. Leave it on for 15 minutes, then wash it off with warm water and gently pat the skin dry before toning and moisturizing as normal.

Note: Both spirulina and kelp powder stain, so be careful not to let the face mask come into contact with white towels or clothes.

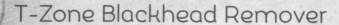

T-Zone Blackhead Remover

for detoxifying

This face mask specifically tackles blackheads and blocked pores in the hard-to-manage T-zone area, which is the forehead, nose and chin. Both the bentonite clay and charcoal are powerful detoxifiers that will help draw out any impurities trapped in the skin. Tea tree essential oil is antibacterial and helps to cleanse the skin. I use gelatine in this recipe as it helps to make a mask that can be peeled off the skin, which helps to pull out blackheads and dirt as it comes off, leaving your skin visibly clearer.

½ teaspoon bentonite clay powder
½ teaspoon activated charcoal powder
1 teaspoon unflavoured gelatine powder
2 teaspoons hot water
1 drop tea tree essential oil

Makes 1 application
Use immediately, or it will become too hard to apply

Put the clay, charcoal and gelatine in a small bowl and stir together. Add the hot water and stir quickly to form a smooth, thick paste, then stir in the drop of tea tree oil. You can add an extra drop or two of hot water if it's too thick to stir.

Using a face-mask brush, apply a layer of the mixture to your T zone straightaway, making sure you avoid the eye area. Leave it on for 15 minutes – no longer – then peel it off and marvel at how clean and clear your skin feels and looks. Tone and moisturize as normal.

Note: Do not let this face mask dry for too long, or it will become too hard to peel off your face. If it doesn't all peel off in one go, rub it off gently using a warm, damp facecloth. Also, charcoal stains, so be careful not to let it come into contact with white towels or clothes.

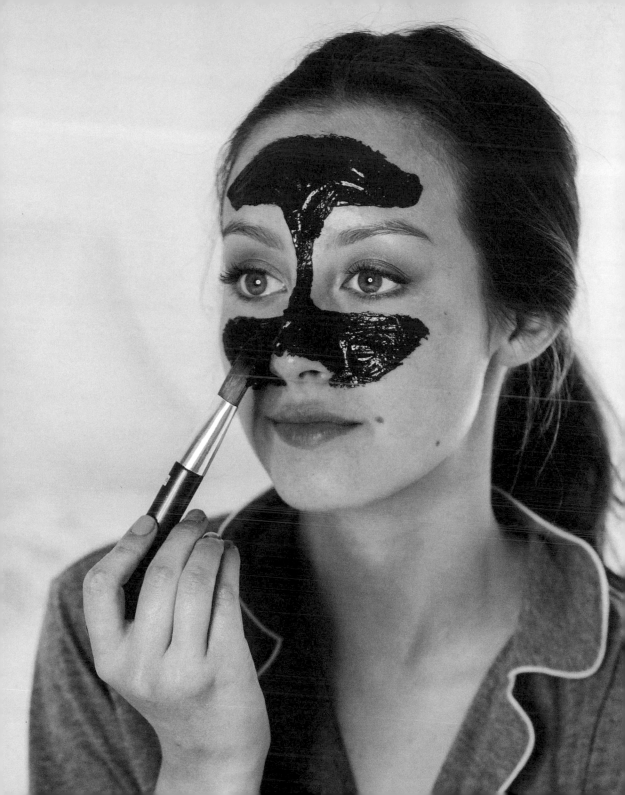

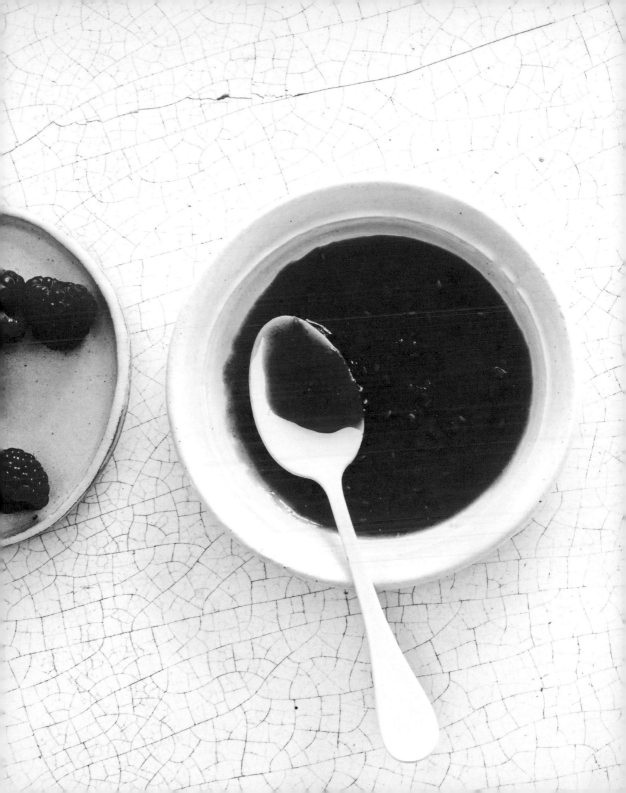

Raspberry Sugar Face Exfoliant

for exfoliating

Raspberries not only taste and smell delicious, but they also contain a large amount of vitamin C, which helps to protect the skin, and the tiny seeds exfoliate the skin, leaving it soft and smooth. The skin on the face is more delicate and sensitive than the skin on the rest of the body, so I always use caster/superfine sugar when making a facial scrub – the larger grains of granulated sugar can be a little too harsh.

4 fresh raspberries
4 teaspoons white caster/superfine sugar
2 drops pure vitamin E oil

Makes 1–2 applications
Keeps for up to 1 day in the refrigerator

Put the raspberries in a small bowl and mash to a pulp using a fork. Stir in the sugar and vitamin E oil.

Apply the scrub to a make-up-free, clean face with your fingertips. Use small, circular motions to gently rub the exfoliant over your cheeks, chin and forehead and around the nose area, but make sure you avoid the eye area because the skin there is too delicate for scrubbing. Do this for a minute or two or until your skin feels refreshed, then wash it off with warm water and gently pat the skin dry. Tone and moisturize as normal.

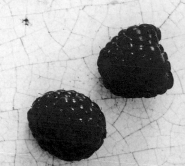

Peachy Glow Facial Scrub

for exfoliating and oily skin

Peaches are packed full of provitamin A carotenoids and vitamin C, plus plenty of other nutrients that are beneficial to the skin. Vitamin C is an antioxidant that protects the skin and can help to slow down the aging process – hurrah! Provitamin A carotenoids encourage the production of healthy skin cells, keeping the skin firm and supple. Peaches also help to regulate oil production on the skin, so this face scrub is good for people with oily skin.

1 slice of fresh ripe peach, approx 2-cm/¾-inch thick
1 tablespoon soft brown sugar

Makes 1–2 applications
Keeps for up to 1 day in the refrigerator

It's best to use a very ripe peach for this recipe because it's much easier to mash up. Put the peach slice in a small bowl and, using a fork, mash it into a fine pulp. Add the brown sugar and stir together.

Apply the scrub to a clean face with your fingertips. Use small, circular motions to gently rub the exfoliant over your cheeks, chin, forehead and around the nose area, but make sure you avoid the eye area. Do this for a minute or two or until your skin feels refreshed, then wash it off with warm water and gently pat the skin dry.

Recipe idea: Peach and Raspberry Breakfast Bowl

When peaches are in season, I just can't help but add them to everything I can. This is a lovely, easy breakfast idea and a great way to use up the leftover peach.

Serves 1

100 g/1 cup granola
2–3 tablespoons natural full-fat Greek yogurt
½ ripe peach, stoned/pitted and cut into cubes
a few fresh raspberries
1–2 teaspoons raw organic honey

Put the granola into a bowl and top it with the yogurt, peach cubes, raspberries and a drizzle of honey, to taste.

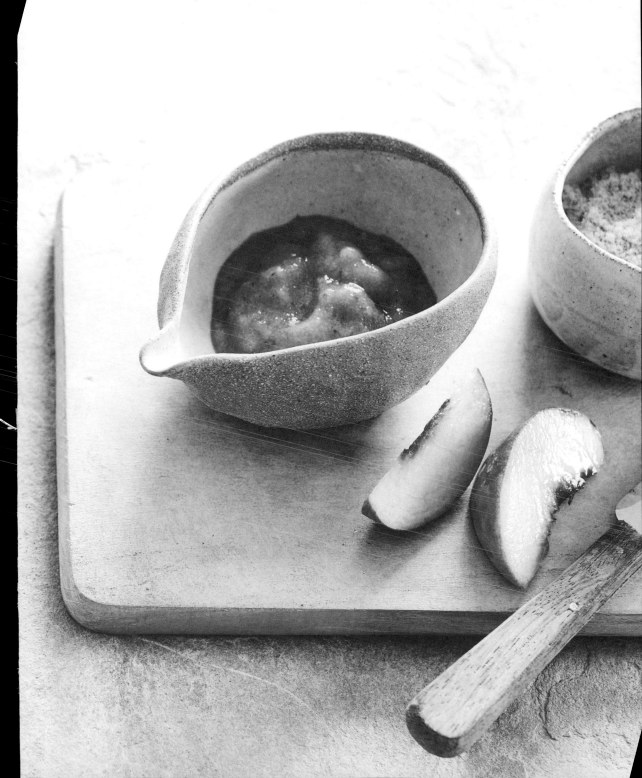

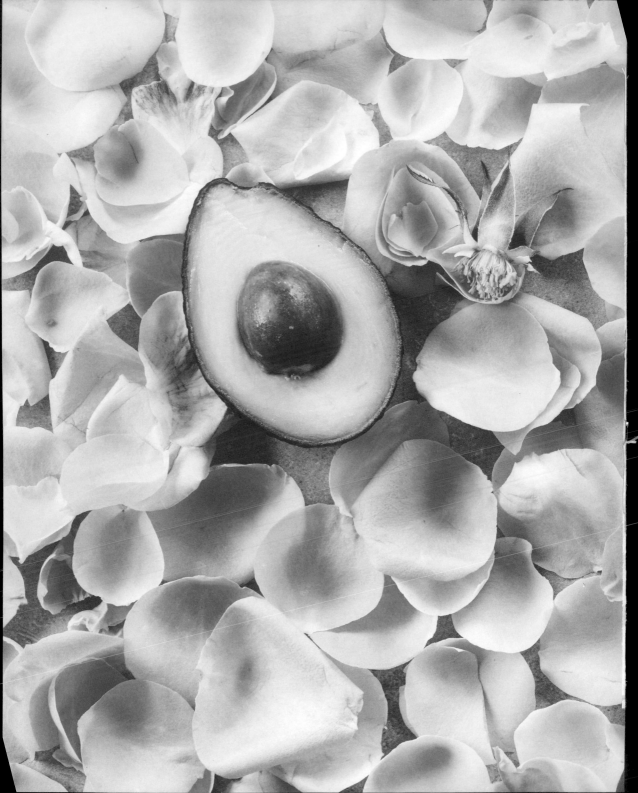

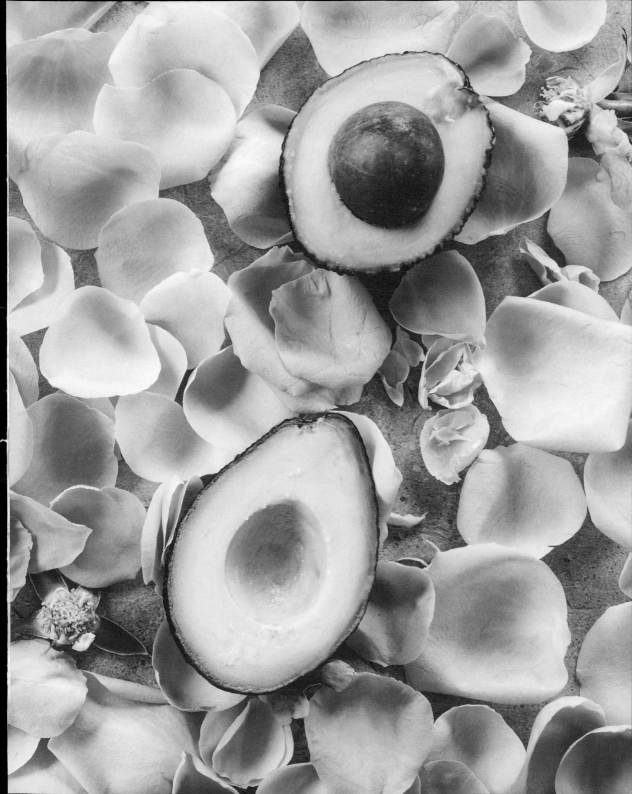

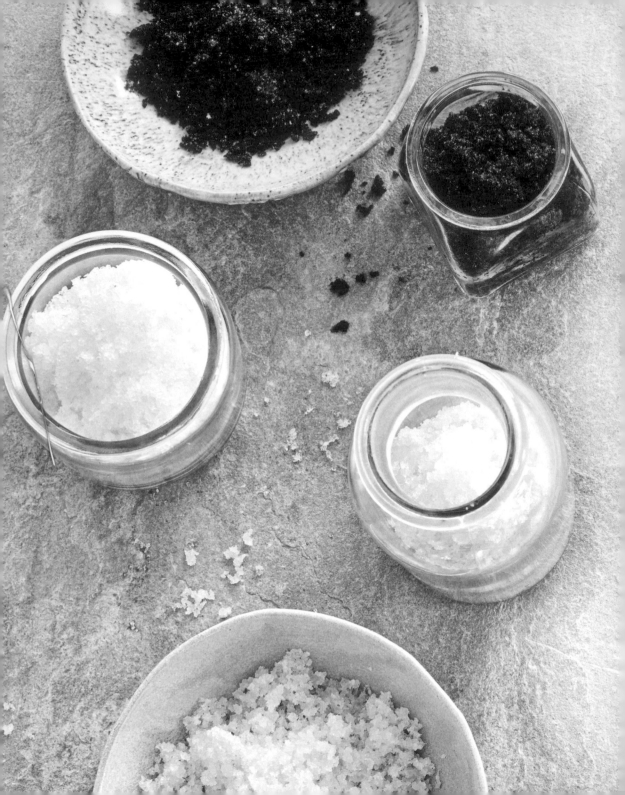

body treatments

Exfoliation is the key to soft, smooth skin, not just on your face but on your whole body. In fact, exfoliating your body gives you the same benefits as exfoliating your face. It helps clear away dead skin cells and unclogs the pores, resulting in clearer, smoother, healthier skin. Once your skin has been properly exfoliated it leaves a fresh surface for your moisturizer to sink deeper into the skin and nourish more effectively.

I use sugar and dead sea salt as bases for the scrubs, then add in moisturizing oils, such as olive, coconut or avocado oil, to keep the skin soft. Giving yourself an exfoliating scrub also helps circulate the blood flow and can help reduce the appearance of cellulite on those dreaded cottage cheese areas. You can use a facecloth, body brush or just your hands to rub the scrubs in. A body brush works best for a more vigorous circulation scrub.

You'll also find a few relaxing bath soaks, such as my Goddess Rose Milk Bath Soak to make your skin silky smooth or the Muscle-Soothing Bath Soak to soothe aching muscles. It's amazing how we can find what we need in nature to help our bodies look their best, while healing and nourishing at the same time.

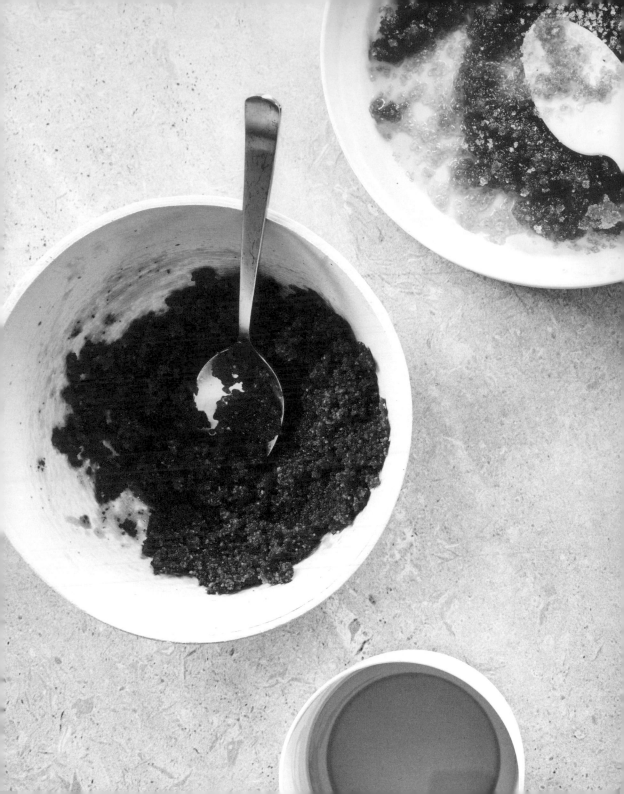

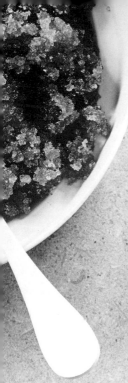

Brown Sugar, Vanilla
+ Olive Oil Body Scrub

normal to dry skin

This is a highly effective natural body scrub that is really easy to make at home – it's a great one to use if you want to scrub away some of that old fake tan. The sugar exfoliates and removes dead skin cells, leaving skin silky smooth. I use raw coconut sugar if my skin is feeling extra dry, as the grains are slightly larger, whereas soft brown sugar will make a finer exfoliator, as the grains are smaller and less harsh on the skin. Olive oil is extremely moisturizing and rich in antioxidants so this scrub will leave your skin soft and well hydrated, and the vanilla smells divine.

150 g/¾ cup soft brown sugar or raw coconut sugar
3 tablespoons extra virgin olive oil
2–3 drops pure vanilla extract

Makes 2–3 applications
Keeps for up to 2 weeks in an airtight container or zip-lock bag – no need to refrigerate

Put all the ingredients in a small bowl and stir together. Transfer the mixture to a small jar with a lid as it makes enough for 2–3 applications.

While you're in either the shower or bath, apply the scrub to wet skin. Using your hands, a washcloth or a body brush, make circular motions to rub the mixture into your skin. Rinse it off with warm water.

Mocha Body Bliss

normal to dry skin

Ground coffee is not only good at gently exfoliating, but it also softens the skin and helps to restore moisture. Pure cocoa is packed full of antioxidants to help nourish dry skin; plus, it makes this body scrub smell so delicious you'll enjoy rubbing it all over yourself. I like to add brown sugar as an extra exfoliant to get rid of dead skin cells, and the coconut oil adds and locks in moisture to your skin.

100 g/½ cup soft brown sugar
40 g/½ cup ground coffee
1 tablespoon pure unsweetened cocoa powder
4 tablespoons pure organic coconut oil

Makes 2 applications

Keeps for up to 2 weeks in an airtight container or zip-lock bag – no need to refrigerate

Put all the ingredients in a small bowl and mix together. This makes enough for two applications, so you can transfer it into a jar with a lid and keep half for another day.

While you're in either the bath or shower, rub the mixture all over your body for a good 5–10 minutes, using your hands, a washcloth or a body brush, then rinse it off with warm water.

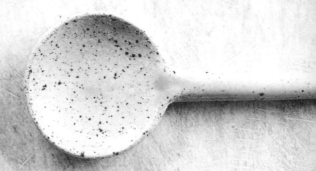

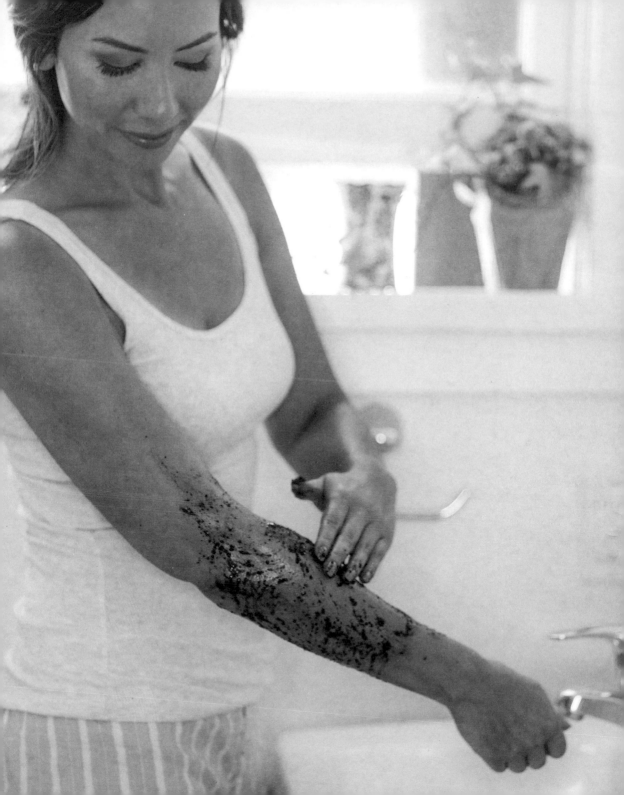

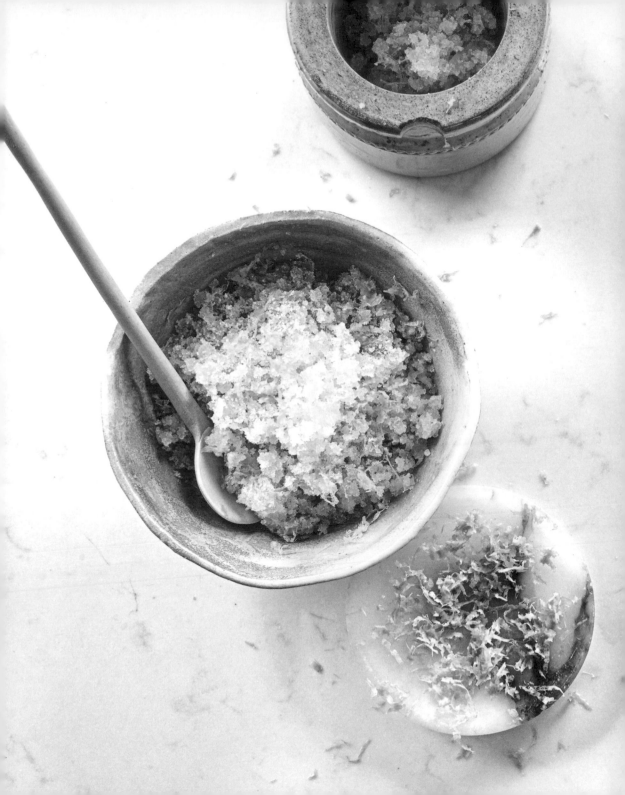

Invigorating Grapefruit + Olive Oil Scrub

normal to dry skin

Grapefruit can do wonders for your skin, especially cellulite-prone areas, because the essential oil contains the concentrate of an anti-inflammatory enzyme called bromelain, which has been known to help break down the fatty deposits that cause the 'cottage cheese' effect on the skin. By regularly massaging and stimulating these areas, you can help to keep the dreaded dimples at bay.

1 tablespoon finely grated grapefruit zest
100 g/ ½ cup white granulated sugar
2 teaspoons fine sea salt
3½ tablespoons extra virgin olive oil
7 drops grapefruit essential oil

Makes 2 applications
Keeps for up to 2 weeks in an airtight container or zip-lock bag – no need to refrigerate

Put all the ingredients in a small bowl and mix together. This makes enough for two applications, so you can transfer it into a jar with a lid and keep half for another day.

Apply the body scrub to wet skin when you are in either the shower or the bath, using circular motions as you rub it into your skin. For increased stimulation to the cellulite-prone areas, use a body brush to help exfoliate the skin and improve circulation. Rinse off the scrub with warm water.

Coffee Berry Power Scrub

cellulite-prone areas

Ground coffee has been known to help reduce the appearance of cellulite if used regularly on problem areas; the coffee grains contain caffeine, which tightens the skin. The secret ingredient in my scrub is coffee berry powder, for an extra-powerful boost of antioxidants. The coffee berry is the fruit that surrounds the coffee bean and it has been named a superfood due to the large amounts of antioxidants and phytonutrients it contains. The coconut oil moisturizes the skin, while the sugar works as an extra exfoliator. Using a dry body brush with this scrub will also help to stimulate the blood flow and circulation.

100 g/ ½ cup soft brown sugar
40 g/ ½ cup ground coffee
4 tablespoons pure organic coconut oil
2–3 teaspoons coffee berry powder

Makes 2–3 applications – I like to double the quantities given above
and keep some in a jar with a lid for a few applications
Keeps for up to 2 weeks in an airtight container or zip-lock bag – no need
to refrigerate

Put all the ingredients in a bowl and mix together.

Stand in a shower or bath tub and before turning on the water, smooth a handful of the scrub onto any areas prone to cellulite. Then, using a dry body brush, rub in small circular motions for a few minutes. Rinse off the scrub with warm water. Repeat 2–3 times a week. Sadly, there is no overnight miracle cure for cellulite, but regularly stimulating the skin can help to reduce its appearance over time, and you'll soon have super-soft and glowing skin.

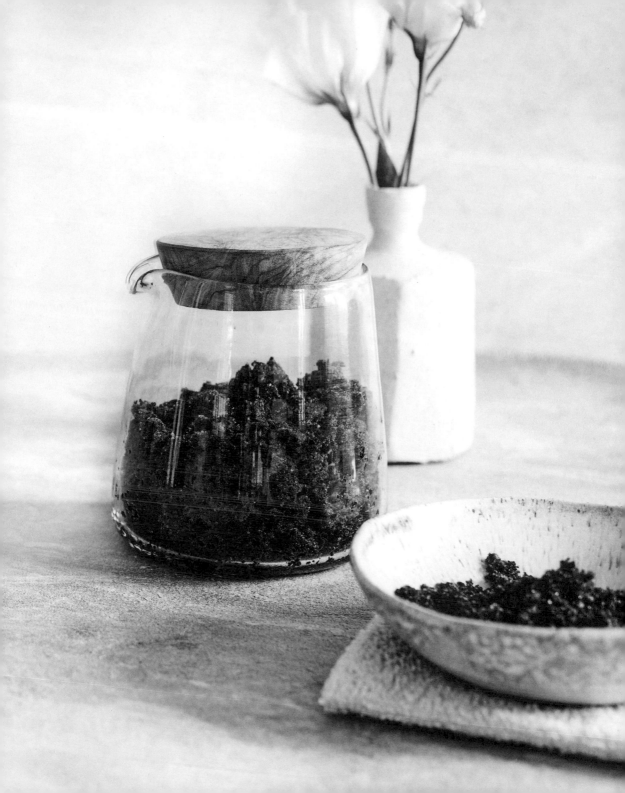

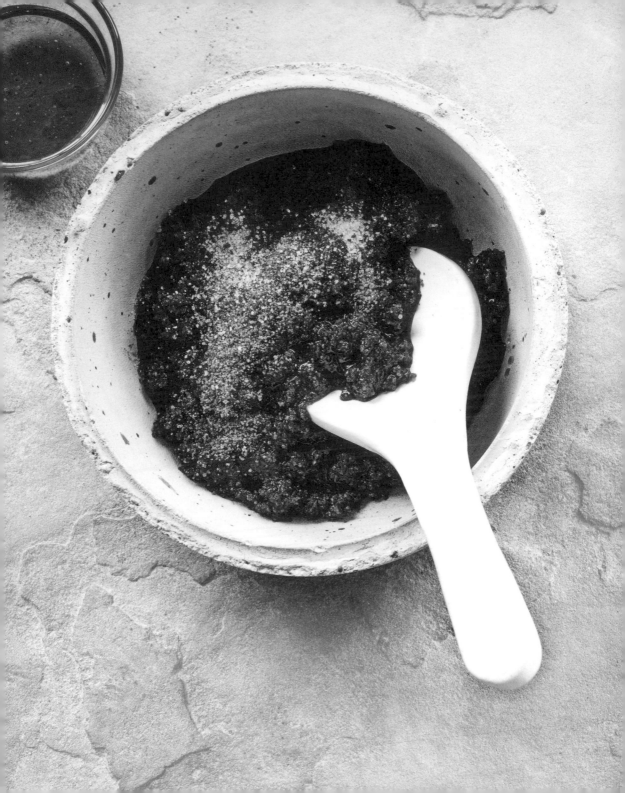

Banana + Cinnamon Sugar Scrub

normal to dry skin

Cinnamon is a wonderful natural ingredient that has been used for centuries in health and beauty remedies. When used on the skin, it acts as an exfoliant and helps to remove dead skin cells; it also has anti-fungal and antibacterial properties, which help to keep the skin clean and clear. Bananas are highly moisturizing and contain potassium and vitamins E and C, which promote healthy, glowing skin.

¼ ripe banana, peeled
1 teaspoon ground cinnamon
1 tablespoon raw organic honey
50 g/ ¼ cup raw coconut sugar or soft brown sugar
50 g/ ¼ cup white granulated sugar

Makes 1 full-body mask and scrub
Use it straightaway, as fresh bananas don't keep very well

Put the banana in a small bowl and mash with a fork. Add the cinnamon, honey and sugars and mix together.

Using your hands, a washcloth or a body brush, use circular motions to rub this divine-smelling body scrub all over your body (apply it to dry skin). Wash it off with warm water and you'll be left with silky, soft skin.

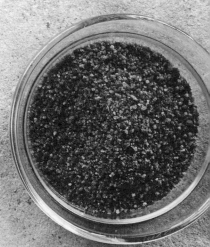

Muscle-Soothing Bath Soak

aching muscles

This bath soak is the perfect way to relax and soothe aching muscles after a long, hard day. Epsom salts has been used for centuries to help relieve sore muscles. It contains large quantities of magnesium and sulphates/sulfates, essential minerals our bodies need, which can be absorbed through the skin while we soak in it. Magnesium relaxes the muscles and helps to regulate muscle and nerve function, while sulphates/sulfates aid the body's detoxification.

500 g/2 cups Epsom salts
5 drops lavender essential oil

Makes enough for one bath
Use immediately

Run a full, hot bath, add the Epsom salts and lavender oil, and swirl the water around to dissolve the salts. Relax in the bath for as long as you can before it becomes too cool, a good 20–30 minutes. This way, you give your body plenty of time to detoxify and then absorb the essential minerals.

I like to use the following body oil recipe to moisturize my skin after this soak.

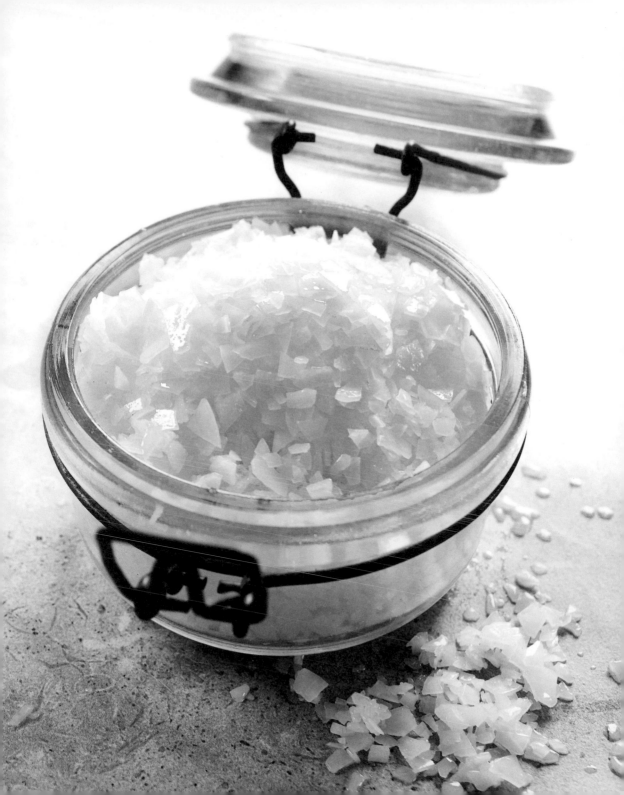

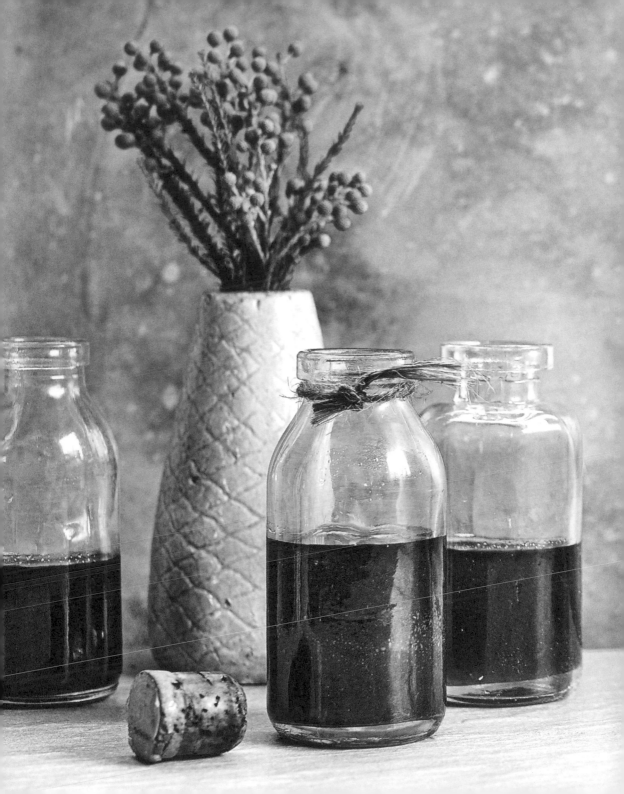

Bedtime Body Oil

normal to dry skin

Avocado oil is one of my favourite oils for slathering over the body because it contains high levels of vitamin E and omega-3 fatty acids to help keep the skin plump and soft. Jojoba oil is a bit lighter and an excellent moisturizer, so blending the two makes it not so heavy. I add lavender essential oil as it helps you relax, while bergamot essential oil has a naturally calming and soothing effect, to settle you into a dreamy sleep at night.

60 ml/¼ cup pure avocado oil
60 ml/¼ cup pure jojoba oil
12 drops lavender essential oil
10 drops bergamot essential oil

Makes 20–25 applications
Keeps for up to 3 months

Pour the oils into a bowl or jug/pitcher, add the essential oils and stir them all together. Pour the solution into a dark bottle with a lid and keep it in your bathroom cupboard for your evening body-oil treat.

Apply to clean, dry skin after a hot bath or shower in the evening.

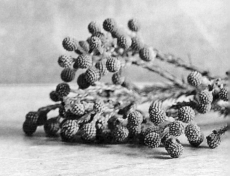

Goddess Rose Milk Bath Soak

normal to dry skin

This bath soak is super-luxurious and a wonderful way to give yourself and your skin a goddess-like treat. The scent of roses has long been used for its natural calming effect and for centuries women have known the benefits of bathing in milk for silky, soft skin. If it's good enough for Cleopatra, it's good enough for us! Milk contains fats and proteins that are absorbed by the skin as you bathe, keeping it well hydrated and moisturized. The rose petals aren't essential but they make your bath look really pretty. Dim the lights and get the candles out, too. You're welcome!

250 g/2 cups organic full-fat milk powder
60 ml/¼ cup pure rosewater
3 drops rose essential oil
a handful of rose petals (optional)

Makes enough for one bath
Use immediately

Run a full, hot bath, add the milk powder, rosewater and rose essential oil, and swirl the water around to dissolve the milk powder and mix everything well. Lastly, sprinkle a handful of rose petals onto the water (if using) and step into a bath made in the heavens.

Relax in the bath for a good 20–30 minutes before it becomes too cool.

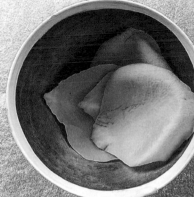

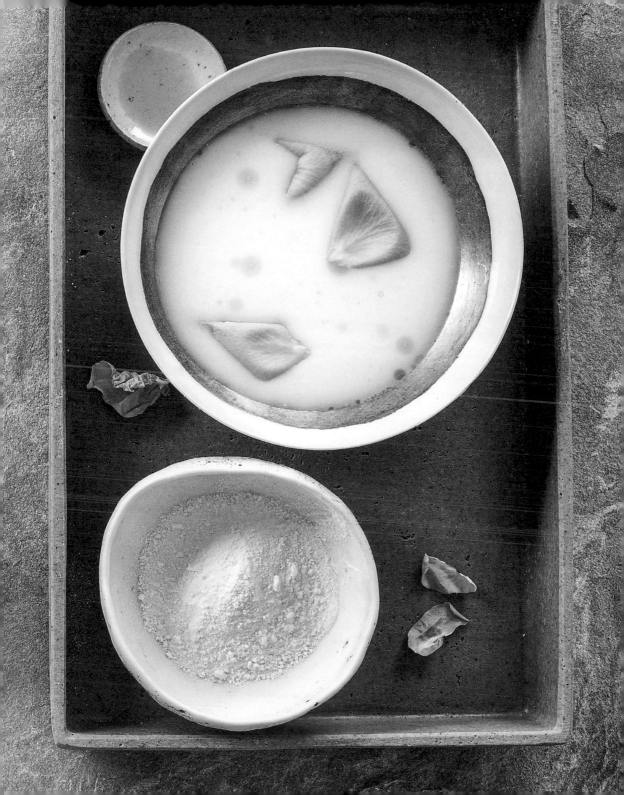

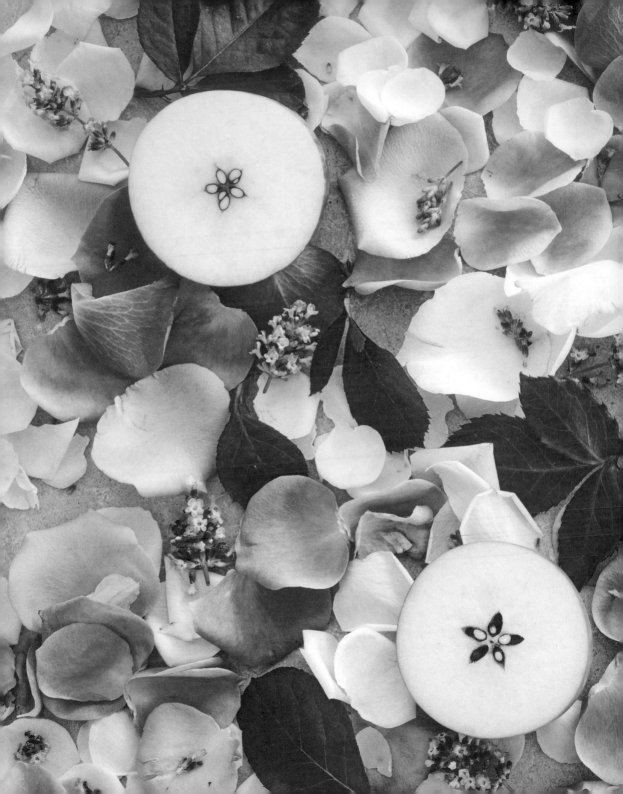

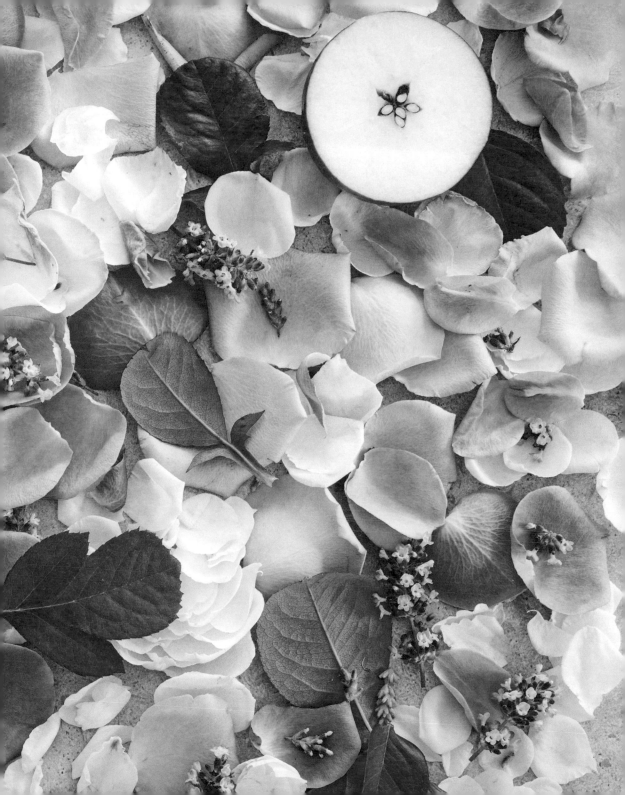

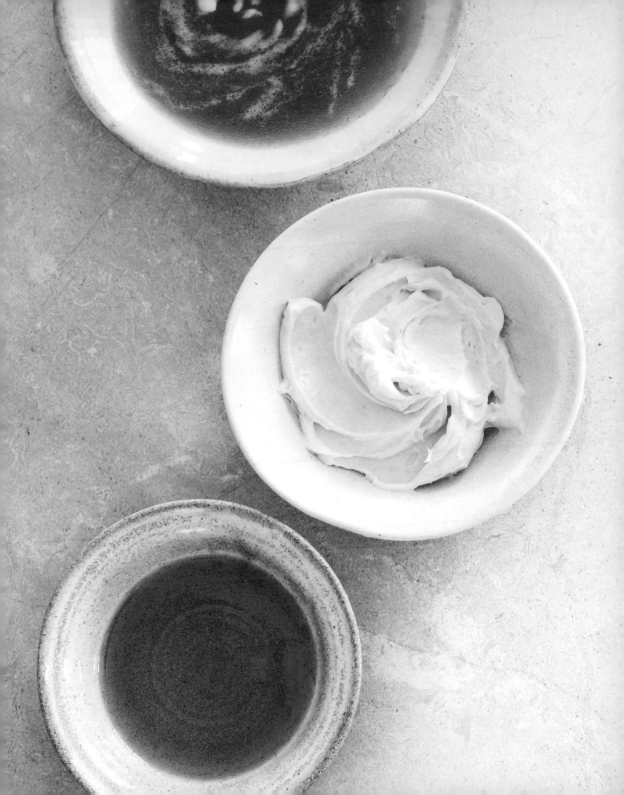

hand + nail treatments

I often find myself imparting my mother's wisdom when talking about beauty. One thing she would always tell me is that your hands will show your age, and that I need to make sure I look after them. Our hands can actually age faster than our faces as there is little fat on the back of our hands and the skin is thin.

The recipes in this chapter are made with naturally nourishing and moisturizing ingredients to keep hands and nails looking and feeling their best. One of my favourite ingredients has to be raw shea butter, your skin's best friend. It's thick, luxurious and full of vitamins and moisturizing natural oils, which absorb beautifully into your hands and nails. I have also included my favourite hand scrubs that I use at home every day. I love to use ingredients like lemons for freshness and removing any stains or strong scents, or lavender for a soothing balm. Sugar is a great natural exfoliant, and using a hand scrub can help you enjoy smoother softer hands, plus it also helps any extra moisturizer to be absorbed more effectively into your skin.

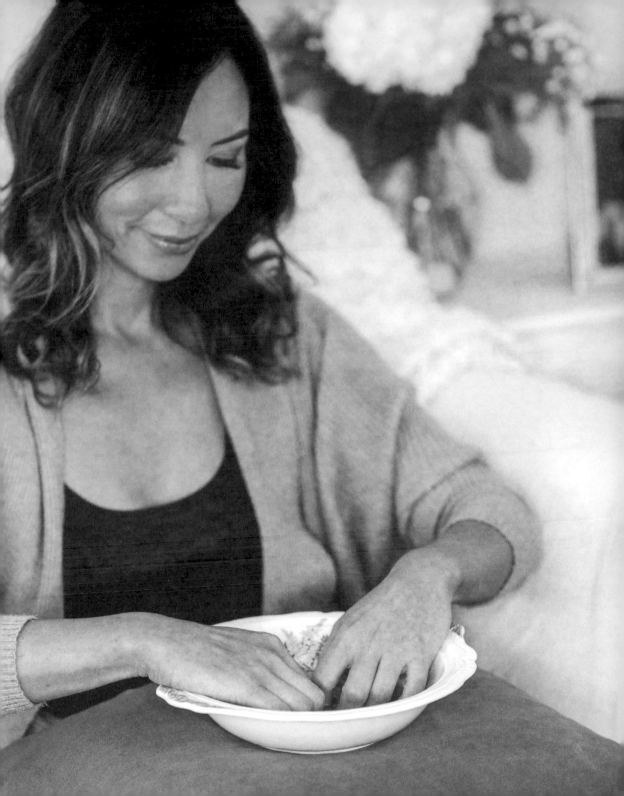

Tea Tree, Lemon +
Olive Oil Warm Nail Soak

for discoloured, brittle or fungus-prone nails

Tea tree essential oil reminds me greatly of my late mother. She studied aromatherapy for years and I'd say this was the essential oil she used the most. It is a powerful natural antiseptic and can help clear up many infections. Olive oil is a natural moisturizer and lemon juice contains a high level of vitamin C, which helps protect the nails, removes stains and encourages stronger nail growth.

1 tablespoon extra virgin olive oil
1 teaspoon freshly squeezed lemon juice
3 drops tea tree essential oil

Makes 1–2 applications – you can also use this on your toenails and feet
Use immediately

I like to warm the oils as I find it more relaxing. First mix all the ingredients together in a small bowl. You can gently heat the mixture in a small saucepan until just warm or, even better, use an essential oil burner. Put a clean dish on top, add the mixture and light a candle underneath to heat it up. This is a great way to heat up small quantities of oils for treatments like this and it also makes the house smell delicious.

Massage the warm mixture into your nails, cuticles and hands, then sit still and relax for 15 minutes. I like to wear vinyl gloves when I've applied this treatment to maximize the effect (as well as ensuring I don't accidentally put oily hands on my furniture). Finally, wash it off and dry your hands well.

Lavender, Sea Salt + Coconut Hand Scrub

all skin types

Dead Sea salt contains more than 20 essential minerals for healthy, strong nails, while acting as a great exfoliant for dry, tired hands. The coconut oil helps to replenish the skin's moisture and also has antimicrobial properties to protect the skin and nails from harmful microbes. This also makes a lovely foot scrub.

3 tablespoons Dead Sea salt
1 tablespoon solid pure organic coconut oil
6 drops lavender essential oil
1 teaspoon crushed dried lavender (optional)

Makes 2 applications
Keeps for up to 2 weeks in an airtight container or zip-lock bag
   – no need to refrigerate

Put all the ingredients into a small bowl and mix together.

Massage the scrub onto your hands and work it all around the nails and cuticles. Leave it on for 5 minutes, then rinse off with warm water and dry your hands. I like to use this while I'm in the bath so I can do my hands and feet at the same time.

Note: This scrub makes a lovely gift and I like to triple or quadruple the quantities given above to make enough for a small jar.

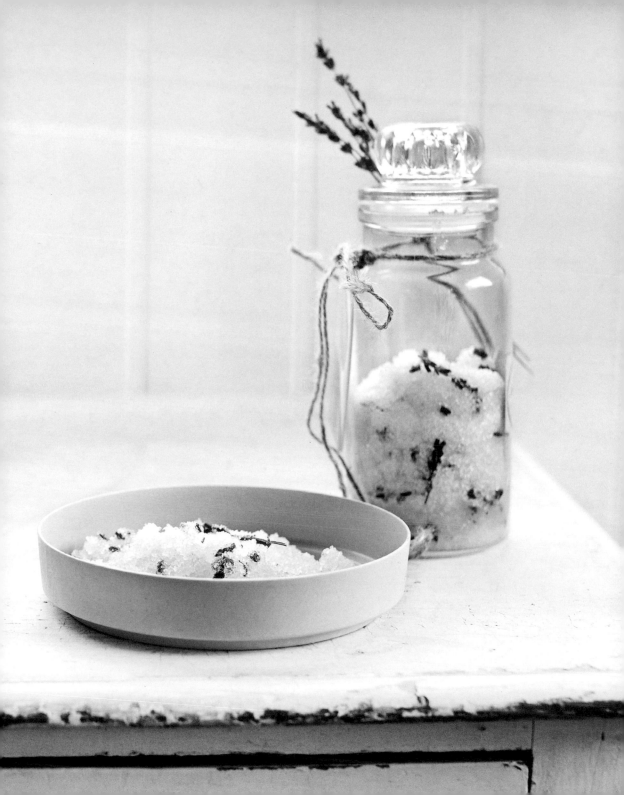

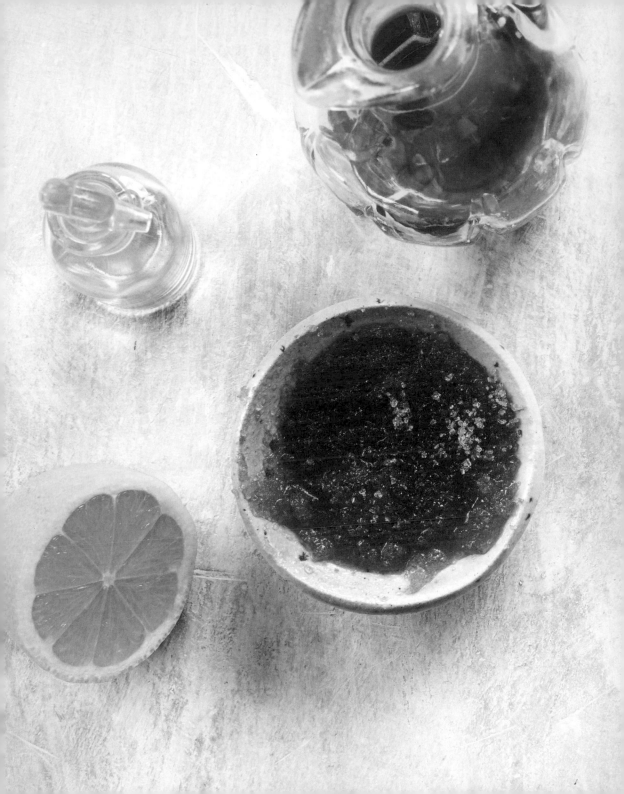

Revitalizing Lemon Sugar Hand Scrub

normal to dry hands

This is the perfect scrub to help refresh dry, aching hands. As a chef, I am constantly washing my hands when dealing with food. I always keep hand cream nearby and I often use this scrub after a day's work to keep my hands soft and refreshed. I love to use lemon as it smells clean and fresh, plus it has plenty of vitamin C to feed and nourish my skin.

100 g/½ cup raw brown sugar (demerara or turbinado)
50 g/¼ cup white caster/superfine sugar
2 tablespoons extra virgin olive oil
freshly squeezed juice of ½ lemon
15 drops lemon essential oil

Makes 4–5 applications

Keeps for up to 2 weeks in an airtight container or zip-lock bag – no need to refrigerate

Put all the ingredients in a small bowl and mix together. Transfer the mixture to a clean jar with a lid.

When you need to use the scrub, take a large tablespoonful and rub it all over your hands. Give yourself a hand massage for about 3–4 minutes before washing it off with warm water and patting the skin dry.

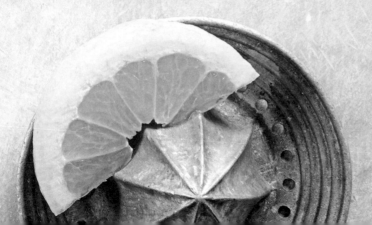

Rose + Lavender Shea Butter Hand Balm

normal to dry hands

This is the ultimate highly moisturizing homemade hand balm. The recipe makes a thick and luscious butter-like cream that your hands will thank you for. Shea butter is packed full of essential fats to keep the skin soft, smooth and protected. I love the soothing combination of rose and lavender, but you can add alternative favourite essential oils instead, if you wish.

40 g/ 1½ oz pure raw shea butter
1 tablespoon extra virgin olive oil
10 drops rose essential oil
8 drops lavender essential oil
5 drops pure vitamin E oil

Makes approx. 55 g/ 2 oz.

Keeps for up to 3 months in an airtight container – no need to refrigerate

Gently melt the shea butter in a double boiler (a small heatproof bowl set over a saucepan of simmering water), or in a microwave on its lowest setting for a few seconds. Once melted, pour it into a small bowl, add the rest of the ingredients and stir together. Put the bowl in the freezer for 10 minutes to help it solidify. Using an electric whisk, beat the mixture until it is fluffy and has turned a lighter shade. You may need to pop it back in the freezer for a few more minutes to help it cool to the right temperature. Once the mixture has been sufficiently beaten, you can transfer it to a clean jar with a lid.

This balm lasts a long time as it is so rich and creamy that you only need a small amount for each application. It melts onto your skin like butter, leaving your hands silky, soft and smelling of roses.

Note: This balm makes a beautiful gift for friends and family, especially when transferred into gorgeous jars, which are easy to find online, with pretty ribbons wrapped around them.

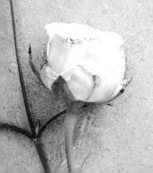
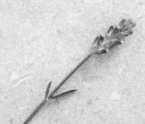
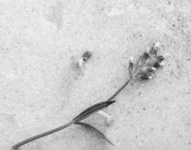

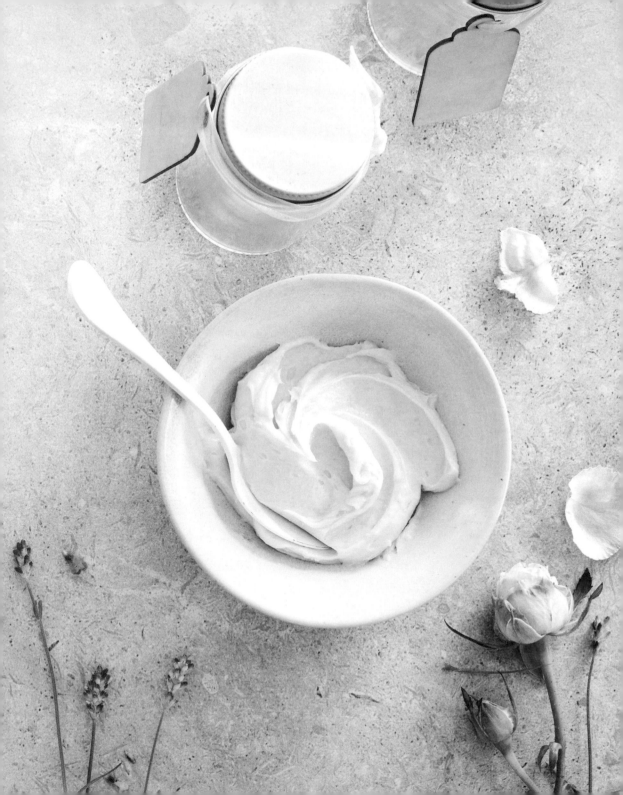

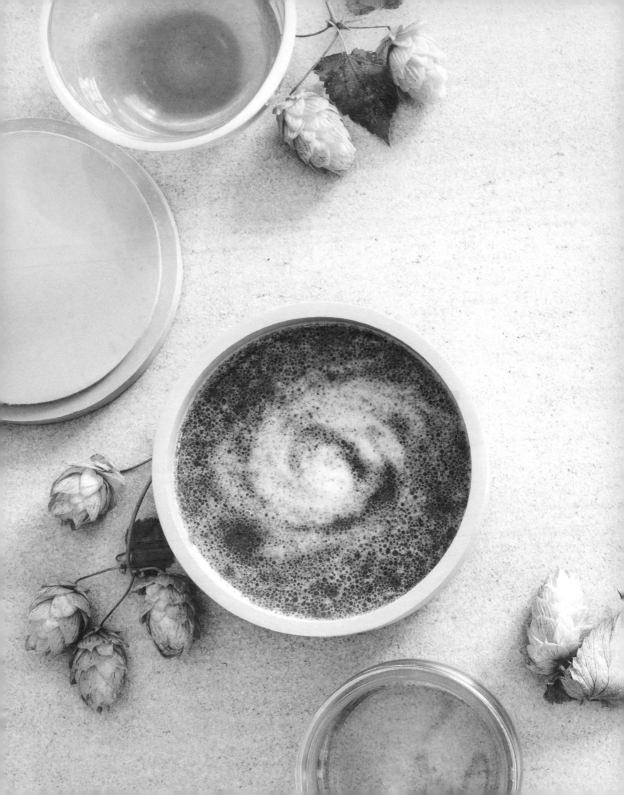

Brittle Nail Soak

brittle nails

Apple cider vinegar helps combat brittle nails because it contains many nutrients, such as iron, calcium, vitamins, potassium and magnesium, which nails need in order to grow strong and healthy. It also contains acetic acid and malic acid, which help prevent nail infections. Beer is not only good for drinking occasionally on a hot summer's day, but it also contains nail-friendly nutrients, such as biotin and selenium, to help keep them strong. The olive oil and vitamin E oil give a natural moisturizing boost.

120 ml/½ cup flat organic dark beer
2 tablespoons extra virgin olive oil
60 ml/¼ cup organic apple cider vinegar
3 drops pure vitamin E oil

Makes 1 nail soak
Use immediately

Put the beer and olive oil together in a saucepan and heat until just warm, making sure it doesn't boil. Remove from the heat and pour the beer and oil into a heatproof bowl that is large enough to soak your fingertips of both hands comfortably, and stir in the apple cider vinegar and vitamin E oil.

Find a relaxing spot to sit down, and place your fingers and nails in the mixture for about 10–15 minutes. After soaking, rinse your hands with warm water and pat them dry. You can use this treatment once or twice a week.

Note: Rub some of the homemade Rose + Lavender Shea Butter Hand Balm (see page 80) onto your nails after the soak to help lubricate and keep them strong.

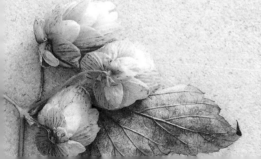

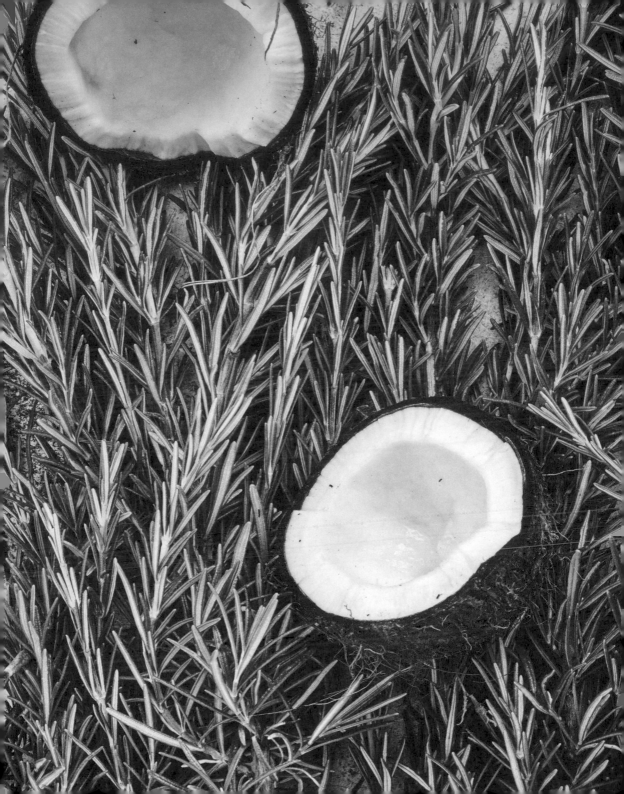

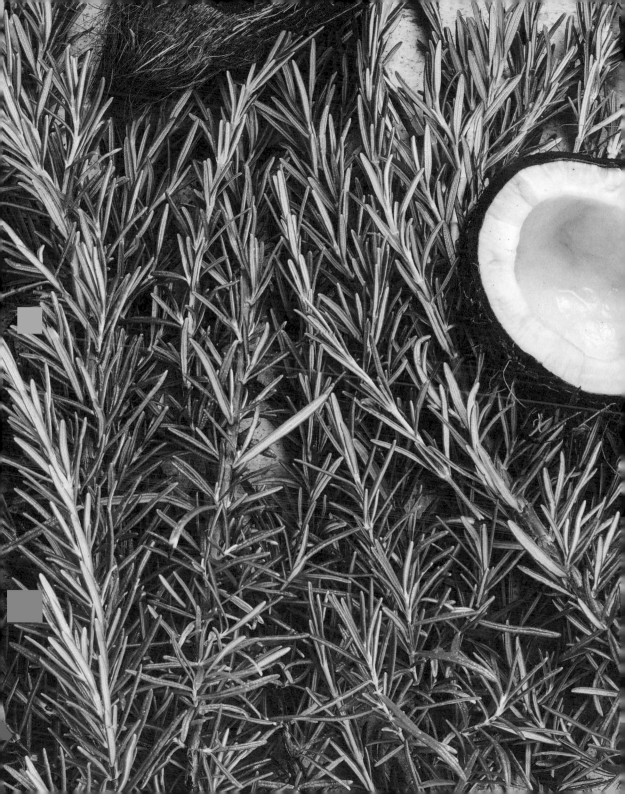

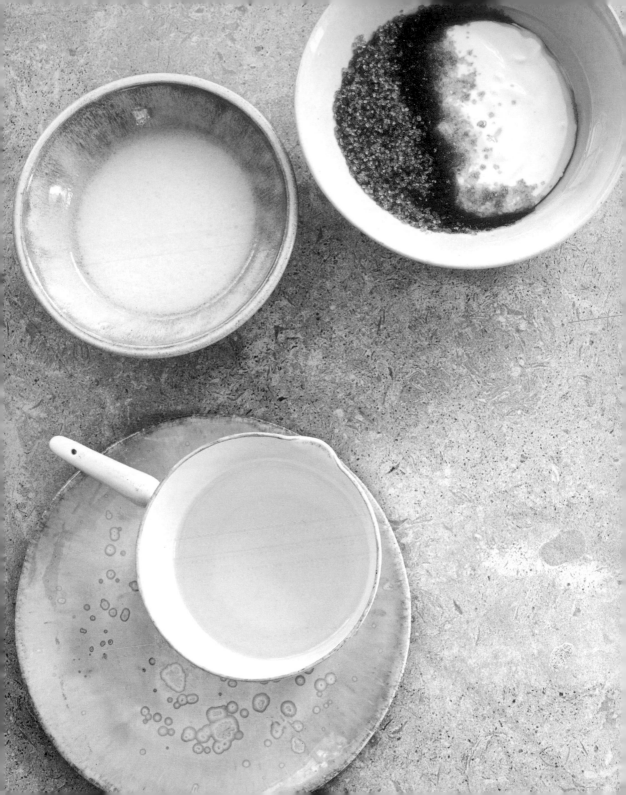

hair masks

We all strive to have thick, luscious locks billowing from our heads. The natural hair masks and hot oil treatments in this chapter will feed and nourish your tresses, leaving hair shiny, thick and smelling divine.

I've included some of my go-to homemade oil treatments, which are designed to give you a healthy scalp, which in turn leads to healthier hair follicles. The scalp has thousands of blood vessels, nerves and sebaceous glands. Sebaceous glands produce oil called sebum, which helps push the hair follicles up to the surface and keeps our skin and hair lubricated.

A great way to keep your scalp healthy is to apply one of the hair treatments and give your head a good massage, using your fingertips, not your nails. This helps to stimulate the blood vessels, encouraging more blood flow, thus nutrients flowing to the hair follicles, and it also helps to gently exfoliate away any dead skin cells or build-up of excess sebum or product stuck in the glands. Your scalp will feel more relaxed, cleaner and the hair at the top of your head lighter. By taking care of your scalp, your hair will grow thicker and stronger.

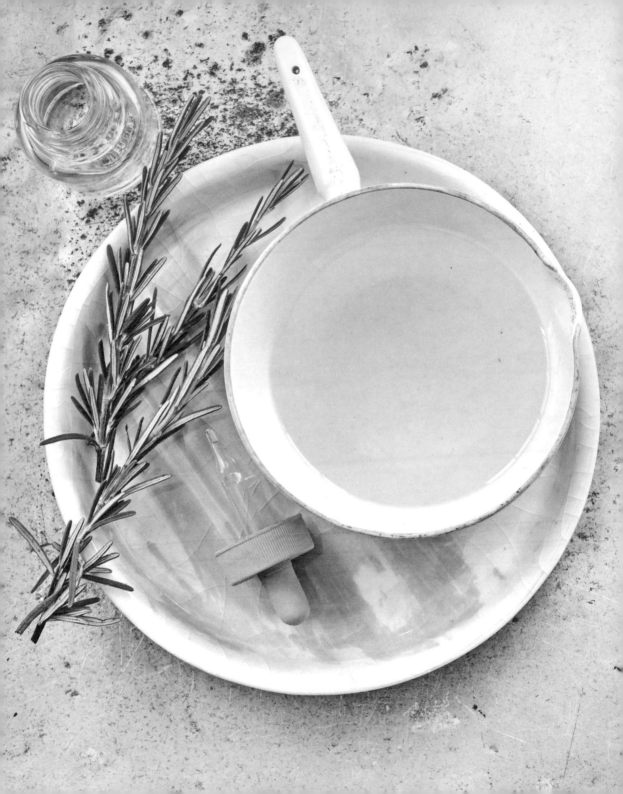

Rosemary + Coconut Hot Oil Stimulant Treatment

for all hair types

Rosemary essential oil is packed full of antioxidants, antibacterial and anti-inflammatory properties, plus it's known to act as a stimulant. The antibacterial and anti-inflammatory properties help to keep the scalp healthy and can aid the treatment of flaky scalps, pimples on the scalp or infections of the hair follicles, which can cause hair loss. Most importantly, the stimulating effect of rosemary oil helps to increase blood flow to the hair follicles, which enables the hair to get the nutrients it needs to grow thicker and stronger. This treatment is even better when you ask someone else to give you a hand massage while applying it.

2 tablespoons pure organic coconut oil
6–8 drops rosemary essential oil

Makes 1 application
Use immediately and repeat weekly

Put the coconut oil in a small saucepan and warm it gently until it melts to a liquid, but do not let it boil. Add the drops of rosemary essential oil and stir together.

Make sure it is not too hot, then gently massage the oil into the scalp and roots of the hair and smooth it over the rest of your hair. Wrap a towel around your head and relax for 15 minutes before washing it out with your favourite shampoo. You can use this hair treatment once a week.

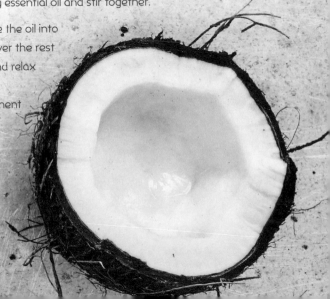

Beer + Honey Wash

for dry to normal hair

Beer has a wealth of nutrients that are excellent for keeping hair thick, strong and shiny. The malt and hops in the beer contain proteins that repair damaged hair, giving it a thicker look; B vitamins stimulate hair growth; sucrose helps keep hair shiny; and, most importantly, biotin is a key nutrient required for healthy hair growth. The egg yolk, olive oil and honey all add extra essential nutrients, plus natural moisture to nourish the hair strands. This recipe is recommended for people with dark to light brown hair. Some dark-coloured beers may leave a slight hue on very light brown or blonde hair after rinsing – though you could try a blonde beer instead.

120 ml/½ cup organic dark beer
1 egg yolk
1 tablespoon raw organic honey
1 teaspoon pure jojoba oil
2 drops sweet orange essential oil

Makes 1 application
Use immediately and repeat once or twice a week

Start by gently heating the beer in a small saucepan until hot. Remove from the heat and leave to cool until just warm. Put the egg yolk, honey, jojoba oil and sweet orange essential oil in a small bowl and mix together. Pour in the cooled beer and mix together well.

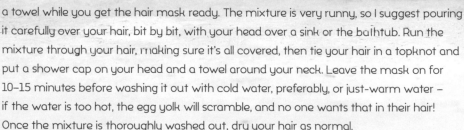

Wash your hair first with your regular shampoo and gently squeeze out any excess water. You can wrap your hair in a towel while you get the hair mask ready. The mixture is very runny, so I suggest pouring it carefully over your hair, bit by bit, with your head over a sink or the bathtub. Run the mixture through your hair, making sure it's all covered, then tie your hair in a topknot and put a shower cap on your head and a towel around your neck. Leave the mask on for 10–15 minutes before washing it out with cold water, preferably, or just-warm water – if the water is too hot, the egg yolk will scramble, and no one wants that in their hair! Once the mixture is thoroughly washed out, dry your hair as normal.

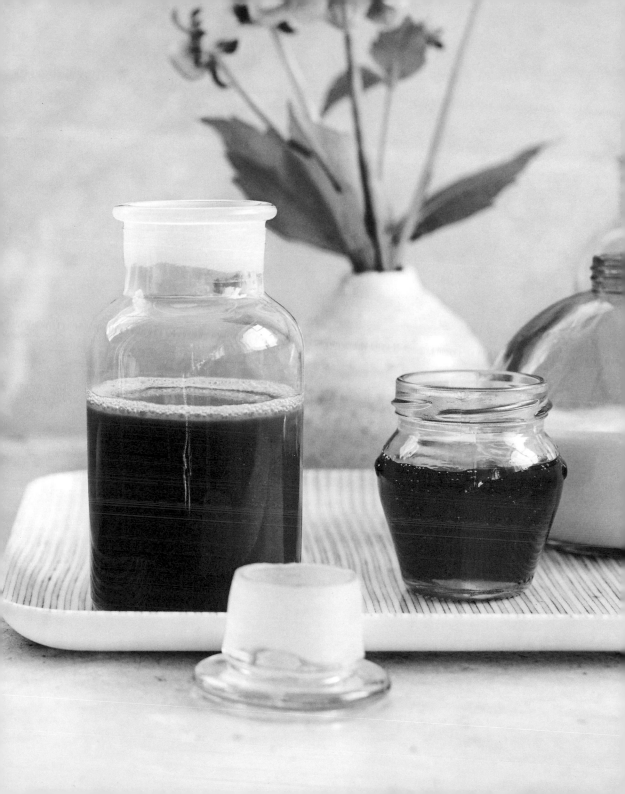

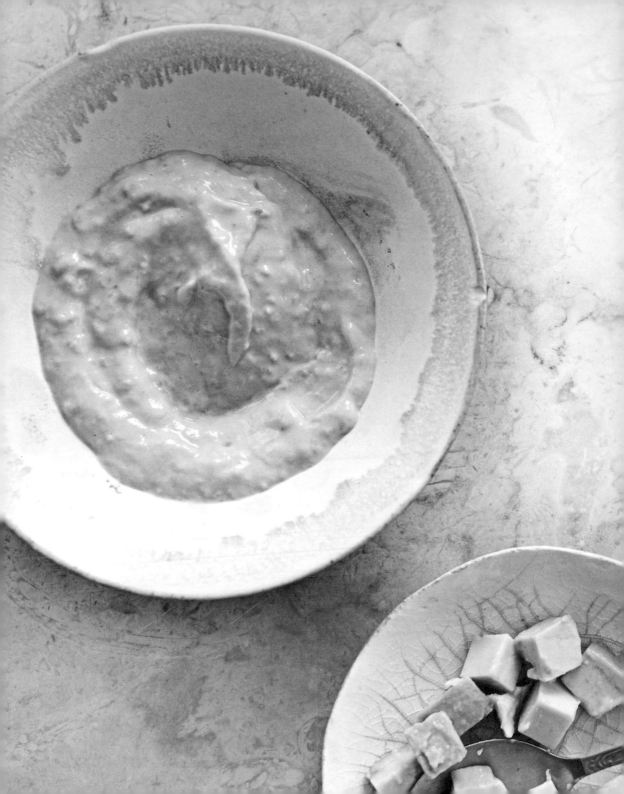

Avocado, Banana + Mayonnaise Hair Mask

for dry and brittle hair

This hair mask is highly moisturizing and luxurious. Avocados are packed full of vitamins and antioxidants that keep hair silky smooth, while bananas contain potassium and antioxidants that help to strengthen weak hair. Mayonnaise is simply made of eggs, which provide protein, and oil, which is moisturizing.

¼ ripe avocado (flesh only)
½ ripe banana, peeled
1 tablespoon organic mayonnaise

Makes 1 application
Use immediately and repeat once or twice a week

Put the avocado and banana in a small bowl and mash with a fork until really smooth, or whizz them together in a small food processor. Stir in the mayonnaise to make a smooth paste.

Using your hands, spread the mixture thoroughly through your dry hair. Leave it on for 30 minutes before washing it off with warm water. Then use a mild shampoo and conditioner to wash your hair as normal.

Note: As all hair types are different, you may or may not need to use conditioner after this hair mask. You can test it out without using any extra conditioner and see how your hair feels once it's dry.

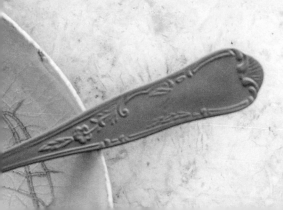

Honey, Coconut + Milk Hair Mask

for normal hair

Milk has been used in skin and hair beauty treatments for centuries. It contains calcium and proteins, which help to restore the natural shine to dull hair. Honey is packed full of essential nutrients and enzymes and has been said to encourage hair growth. Coconut oil has antibacterial and anti-fungal properties to keep the hair and scalp healthy.

½–1 cup/120–250 ml full-fat milk
   (depending on the length
   of your hair)
2 tablespoons raw organic honey

1 tablespoon pure organic coconut oil

Makes 1 application
Use immediately and repeat once or twice a week

Put all the ingredients into a small saucepan and, stirring together, gently heat until just warm enough to touch. If it's too hot, leave it to cool down until it reaches body temperature.

Lean over a sink or bathtub and carefully pour the milk mixture slowly over your hair, massaging it into all the strands so the hair is completely covered. Squeeze out any excess liquid, then tie the hair up in a topknot and put a shower cap on your head and a towel around your neck in case it drips. Leave the mask on for 15–20 minutes, then wash it out with warm water. Shampoo and condition as normal.

Note: As all hair types are different, you may or may not need to use conditioner after this hair mask. You can test it out without using any extra conditioner and see how your hair feels once it's dry.

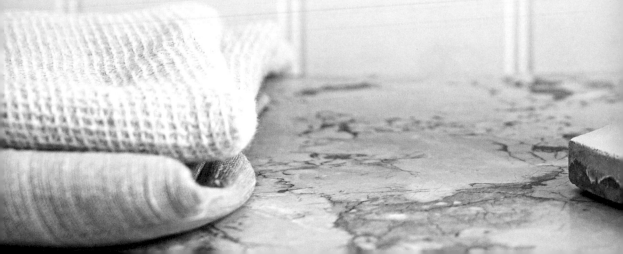

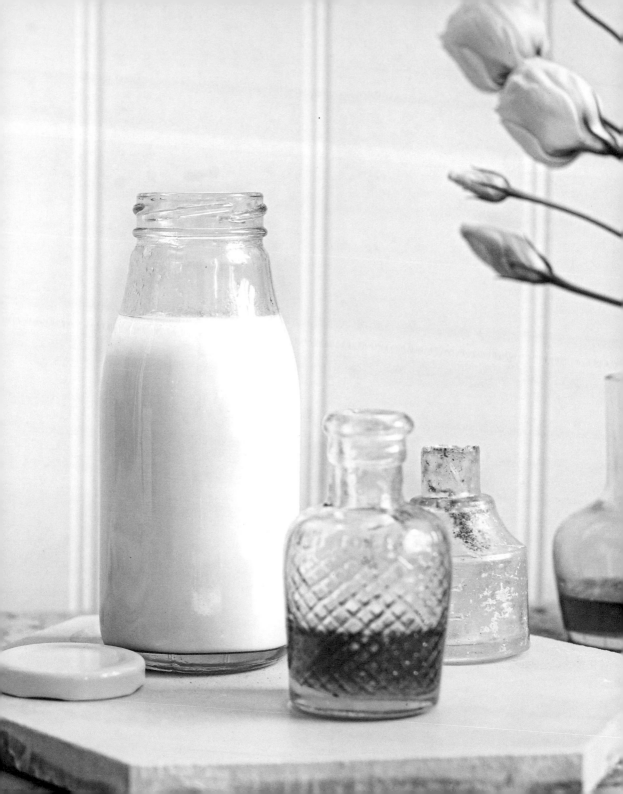

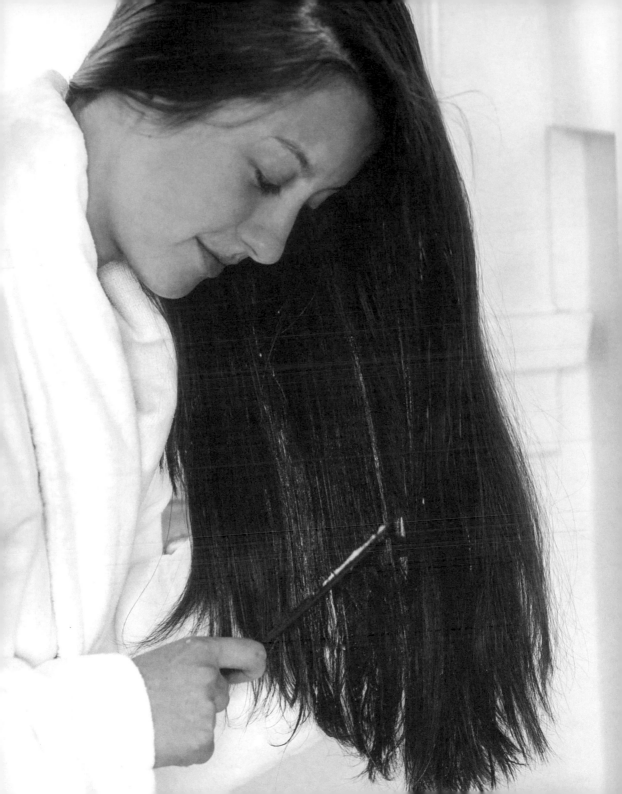

Jojoba Conditioning Scalp + Hair Mask

for dry or damaged hair

This treatment works wonders on dry or damaged hair. Jojoba oil is actually very similar to the oil produced by our skin, making it widely used in beauty products. It contains important minerals, such as copper, zinc and silicon, plus moisturizing vitamin E, and has been known to help promote hair growth by cleaning away excess sebum and moisturizing the scalp and hair follicles without leaving a heavy residue on the hair.

1 tablespoon pure jojoba oil
2 tablespoons natural full fat Greek yogurt
50 g/¼ cup brown demerara/turbinado sugar

Makes 1 application
Use immediately and repeat once a week

Put all the ingredients in a small bowl and mix together to make a paste.

Using your hands, smooth the paste over your hair, starting at the top of your head and then working it through to the ends of your hair. Massage your scalp really well to work the product in. Tie up your hair, cover your head with a shower cap and leave the mask on for 30 minutes. Wash it off with warm water, then shampoo and condition as normal.

Strawberry + Egg White Hair Mask

for greasy hair

If you have greasy hair, it simply means that the sebaceous glands on your head are producing large amounts of oil, which makes your hair greasy. Using harsh, chemical-based shampoos to control this can sometimes have the opposite effect and dry out the scalp, making the glands produce even more oil. Strawberries are a fantastic fruit packed full of the right vitamins and minerals to help clean the scalp and gently balance oil production. Egg white contains less fat than the yolk, but it is packed full of protein to help keep the hair protected, strong and shiny.

100 g/1 cup strawberries, hulled and washed
1 egg white

Makes 1 application
Use immediately and repeat once a week

Blend the strawberries in a small food processor or with a hand-held stick blender until they become a fine, smooth pulp. Put the egg white in a separate bowl and whisk until foamy, then stir in the strawberry pulp.

Apply the mask to wet hair, starting at the top of your head and smoothing it all the way through to the ends of your hair. Tie up your hair, put a shower cap on and leave the mask on for 30 minutes. Thoroughly rinse it off with cold water, making sure you have washed out all of the small strawberry seeds. Do not use hot water to rinse this mask out otherwise the egg white will scramble in your hair. Finally, use a mild shampoo to wash and then condition your hair as normal.

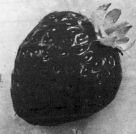

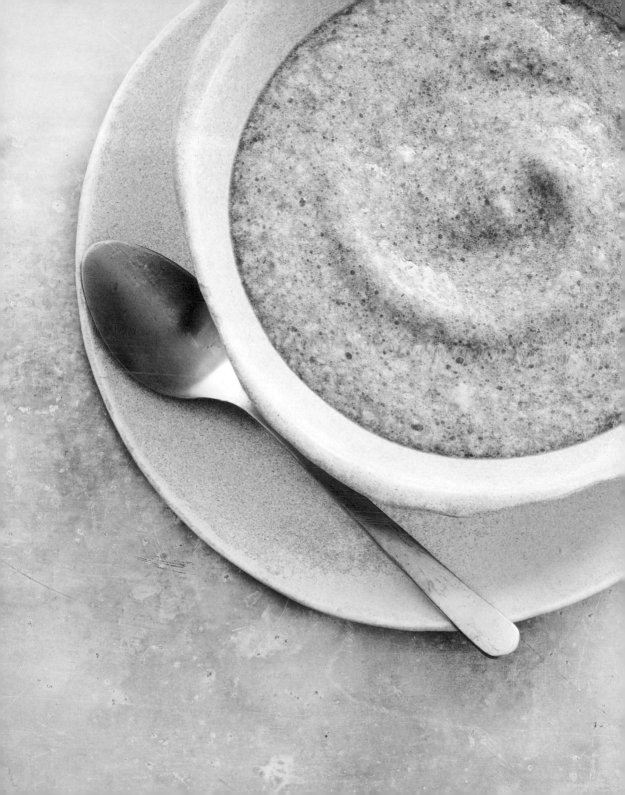

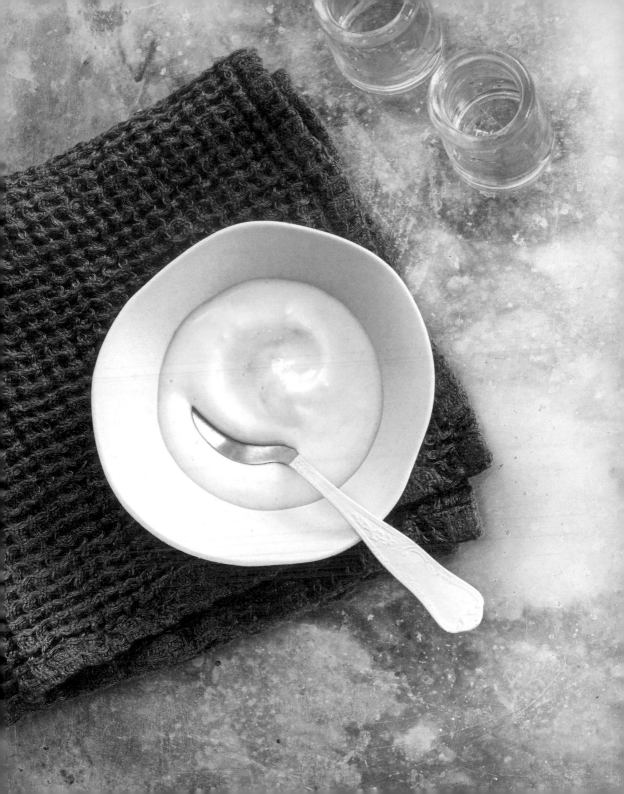

Shea Butter Split End Rescue

for dry or damaged hair

Shea butter acts as a deep conditioner for dry hair. It also works wonders in keeping split ends at bay, by creating a protective coating around the shaft of the hair to keep it strong and healthy.

1 tablespoon pure raw shea butter
1 tablespoon pure organic coconut oil
1 tablespoon pure jojoba oil
2–3 drops essential oil of your choice (optional)

Makes 1 application
Use immediately and repeat once a week

Melt the shea butter and coconut oil together, either in a double boiler (a small heatproof bowl set over a saucepan of simmering water), or in a microwave on its lowest setting for a few seconds. Once melted, put the bowl in the freezer for 10 minutes so it starts to cool down and solidify. Add the jojoba oil and any essential oil you may want to use, then, using an electric whisk, beat until it becomes soft and fluffy.

Apply the mask to the ends of dry hair using your fingers or a comb. Tie up your hair and leave the mask on for 30 minutes. Using a mild shampoo, wash and condition your hair as normal.

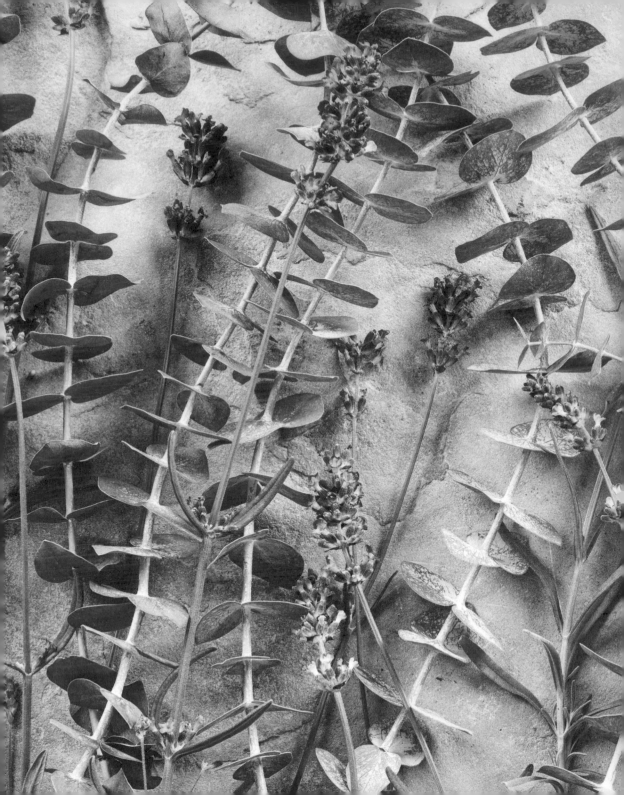

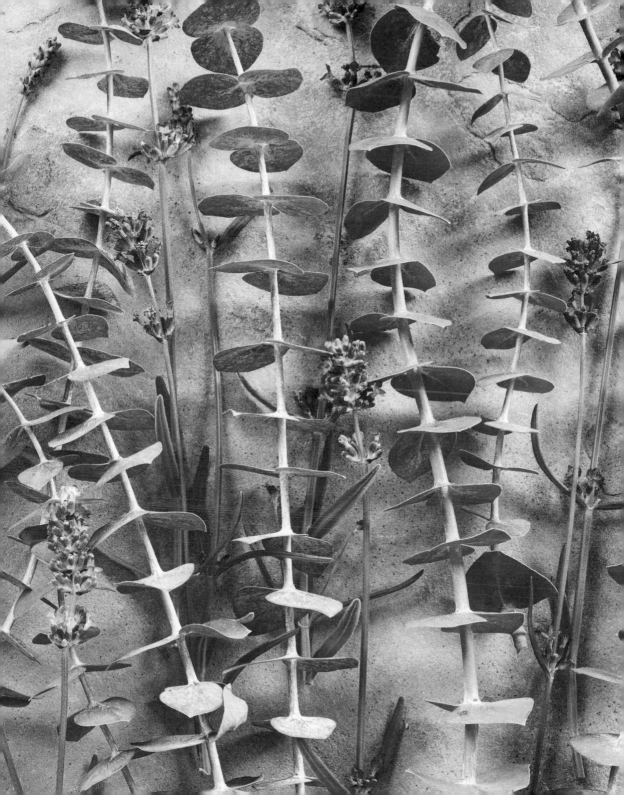

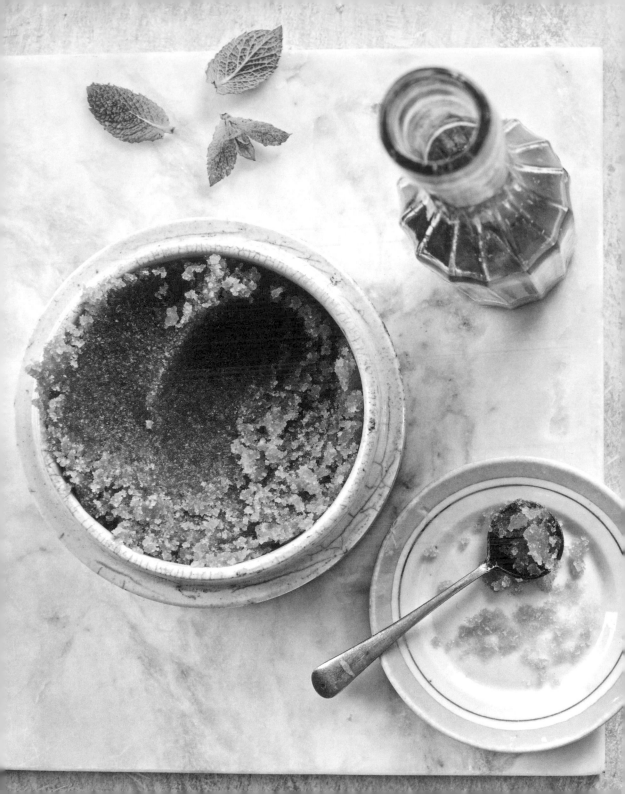

foot treatments

There is nothing better than a relaxing foot soak and rub at the end of a long day. In fact, in Asia, having a foot massage is considered a highly important part of your wellness routine, which stems from the ancient healing art of reflexology.

If you're on your feet all day, you'll be more prone to cracked heels and hard skin due to the pressure. I would start by having a foot bath or soak, then treating your feet to a homemade scrub to exfoliate dead skin. You can also use a pumice stone to help get rid of hard skin on certain parts of your feet. To finish off, use one of my moisturizing foot balms or rubs and slather plenty on your feet before you go to bed. Moisturizing after you've scrubbed or exfoliated will help the natural oils sink deeper into your skin.

Make having a foot bath and massage a regular part of your beauty routine, then not only will you have prettier feet, but you'll also notice the overall health benefits of taking the time to relax and treating your feet with care.

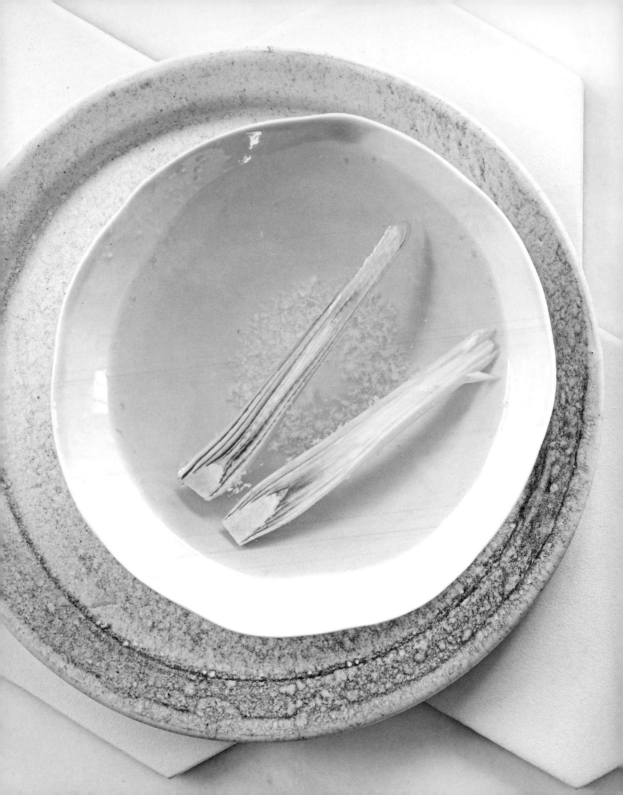

Ginger, Lemongrass + Tea Tree Oil Foot Soak

for treating athlete's foot

Tea tree oil is one of nature's most powerful antiseptics and has been known to be an effective treatment for athlete's foot and other fungal infections. Ginger is known for its detoxifying properties, and lemongrass has antibacterial properties, while the coconut oil provides some added moisture. You can use this treatment even if you don't have any foot infections, as it's a great preventative and good for keeping toenails clean and healthy.

5-cm/2-inch piece of fresh ginger, peeled and grated
2 stalks lemongrass, smashed lightly
1 heaped teaspoon pure organic coconut oil
15–20 drops tea tree essential oil

Makes 1 treatment
Use immediately and repeat 2–3 times a week

To extract the most benefits from the ginger and lemongrass, put them in a saucepan with 950 ml/scant 4 cups of water and bring it to the boil, then turn off the heat to let it steep and cool down.

When you are ready to have a relaxing evening foot soak, pour the ginger and lemongrass water through a sieve/strainer into a foot bowl and discard the bits (or leave them in if you wish). Pour enough hot or warm water into the bowl to cover your feet right up to the ankles. Add the coconut oil and tea tree essential oil and swirl the water around to mix well. Submerge your feet in the bowl and let them soak for 20–30 minutes. You can top up the bowl with more hot water if it begins to get too cool. Dry your feet well, especially between the toes.

Lavender + Oat Relaxing Footbath

for tired and dry feet

This footbath is ideal to have just before bedtime because lavender is a natural relaxing agent and can help get you ready for a deep, restful night's sleep, which is essential for all natural beauty regimes. Oats are a perfect soothing ingredient for dry, chapped skin and help to soften and exfoliate away dead skin cells.

95 g/1 cup rolled oats
8–10 drops lavender essential oil

Makes 1 treatment
Use immediately and repeat 2–3 times a week

Fill a foot bowl with enough hot or warm water to submerge both feet up to the ankles. Simply add the oats and lavender essential oil to the water and stir around for a couple of minutes until the water has turned milky.

Place your feet in the bowl and sit back and relax for 20 minutes. You can top up the bowl with more hot water if it begins to get too cool. I like to give my heels a gentle scrub with a pumice stone at the end of the soak to help keep them smooth. Pat your feet dry and rub a little of your favourite moisturizer or olive oil into your feet to keep them extra soft.

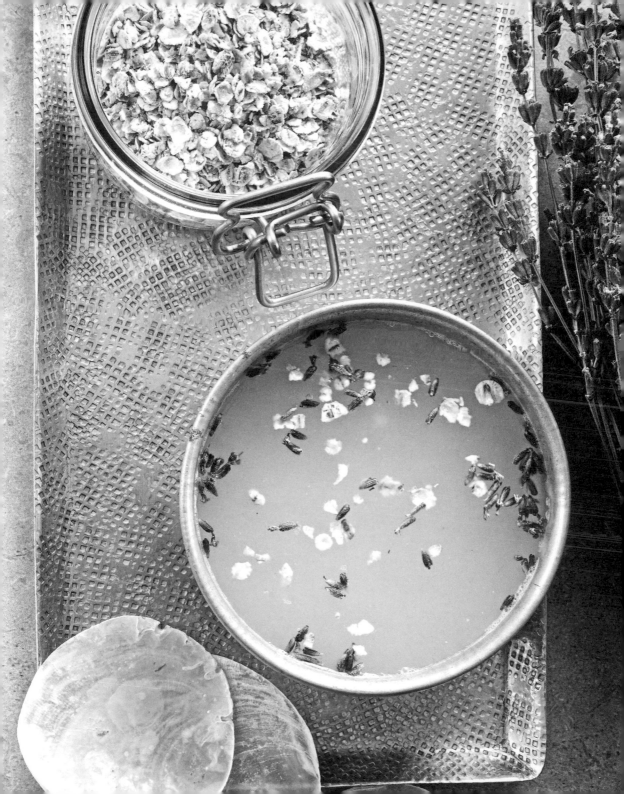

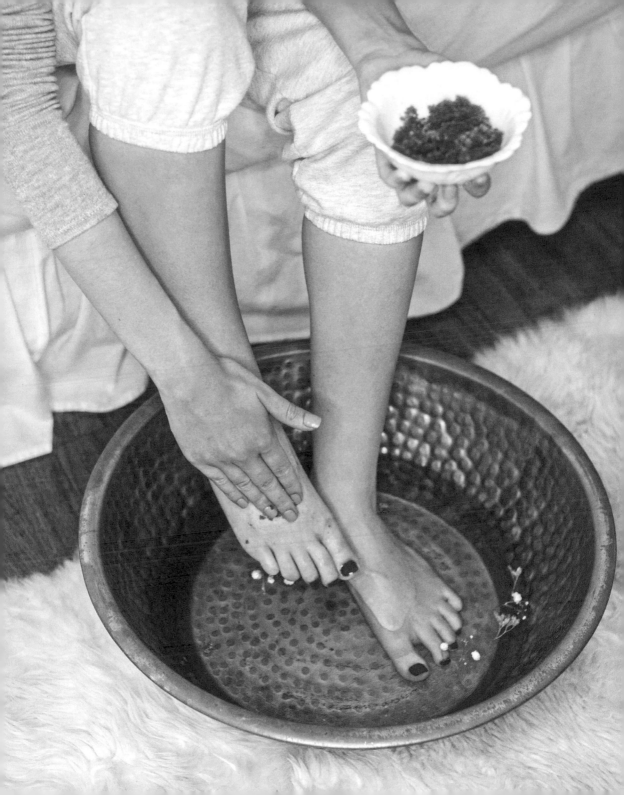

Peppermint + Eucalyptus Foot Scrub

for tired, aching feet

This refreshing and revitalizing foot scrub is for tired and sore feet. I like to use it on my feet after soaking them in one of the footbaths, or at the end of a long, hot soak in the bath. Peppermint essential oil helps to purify the skin, while the eucalyptus essential oil has powerful antibacterial and anti-fungal properties, and also helps relieve aching muscles.

100 g/½ cup soft brown sugar
3 tablespoons extra virgin olive oil
5 drops peppermint essential oil
5 drops eucalyptus essential oil

Makes 2 applications
Keeps for up to 2 weeks in an airtight container or zip-lock bag – no need to refrigerate

Put all the ingredients in a small bowl and mix them together.

After soaking your feet – either in a footbath or after bathing in the tub – simply rub and massage the mixture into your wet feet for a good 5 minutes, or, even better, have someone else do it for you. Wash the scrub off with warm water and pat your feet dry. It's the perfect way to give your feet a treat after a tiring day, and they will smell gorgeously fresh for a long time afterwards.

Note: It is not recommended to use eucalyptus essential oil when pregnant, or if you have high blood pressure or suffer from epilepsy.

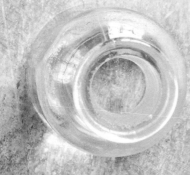

Cocoa Butter Cracked Heel Balm

for dry, cracked heels

If you stand on your feet all day, you're likely to suffer from dry, cracked heels. This is a very healing balm: the honey and aloe vera help to heal the cracks and prevent any infections, while the cocoa butter and coconut oil have a deeply moisturizing effect. This balm is also great for minimizing the appearance of stretch marks.

25 g/1 oz grated raw cocoa butter
3 tablespoons pure organic coconut oil
1 tablespoon raw organic honey
1½ tablespoons pure aloe vera gel

Makes 30–40 applications (115 g/4 oz)
Keeps for 3–4 weeks in the refrigerator in a jar with a lid

Using a double boiler (a small heatproof bowl set over a saucepan of simmering water), or in a microwave on its lowest setting for a few seconds, gently melt the cocoa butter and coconut oil together. Remove from the heat and place the bowl in the freezer for 10 minutes to speed up the chilling process. Add the honey and aloe vera gel. Using an electric whisk, beat together until fluffy. If it's not solidifying, put the bowl back in the freezer for a couple of minutes to get it to the right temperature, then beat again for a few seconds. Transfer the mixture to a clean jar with a lid.

You can apply this balm to your cracked heels every night before bed, and wear socks to protect your bedsheets from grease stains.

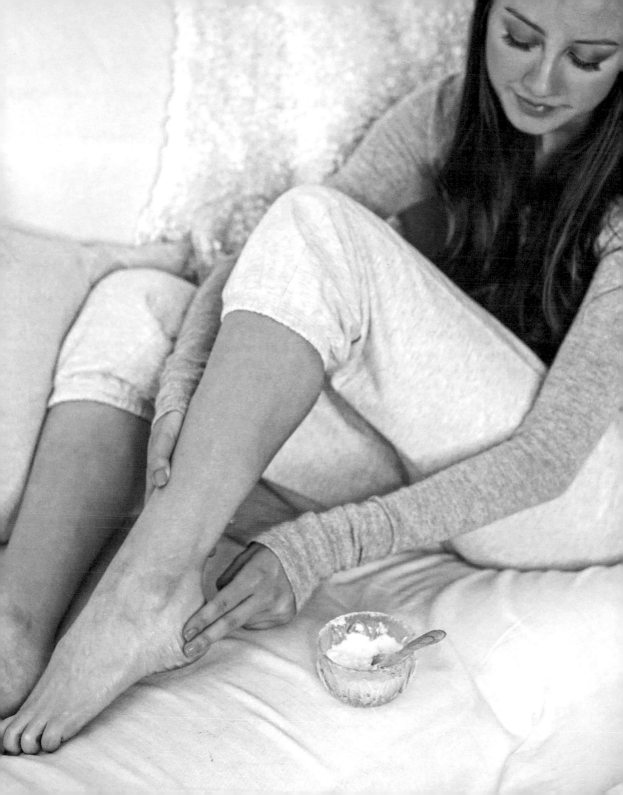

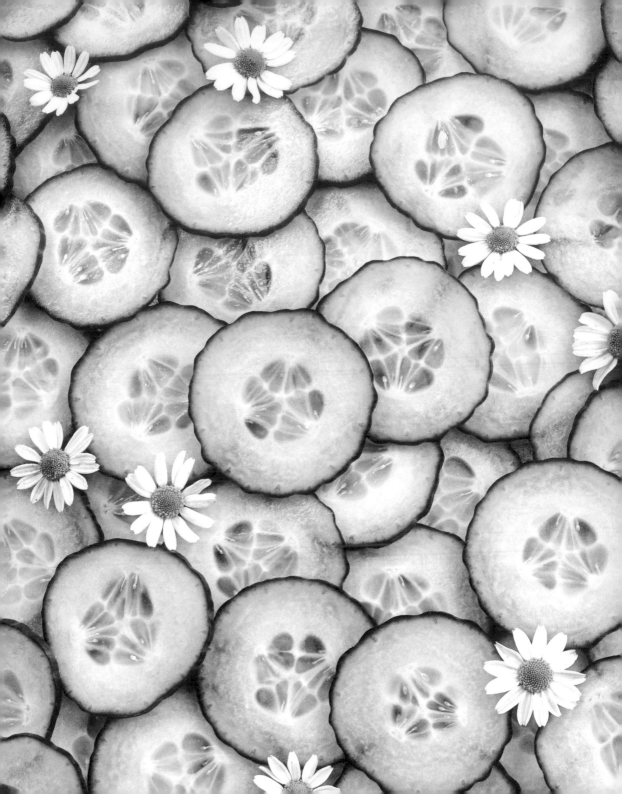

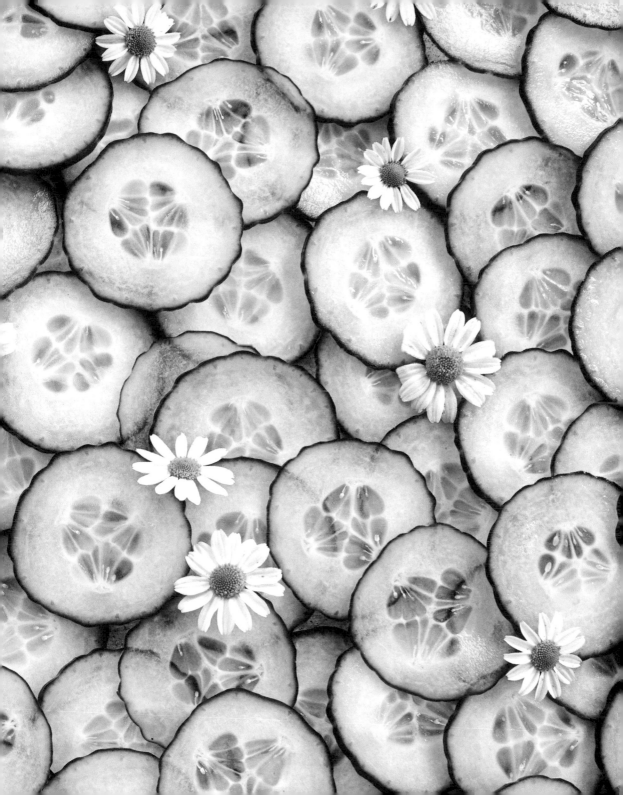

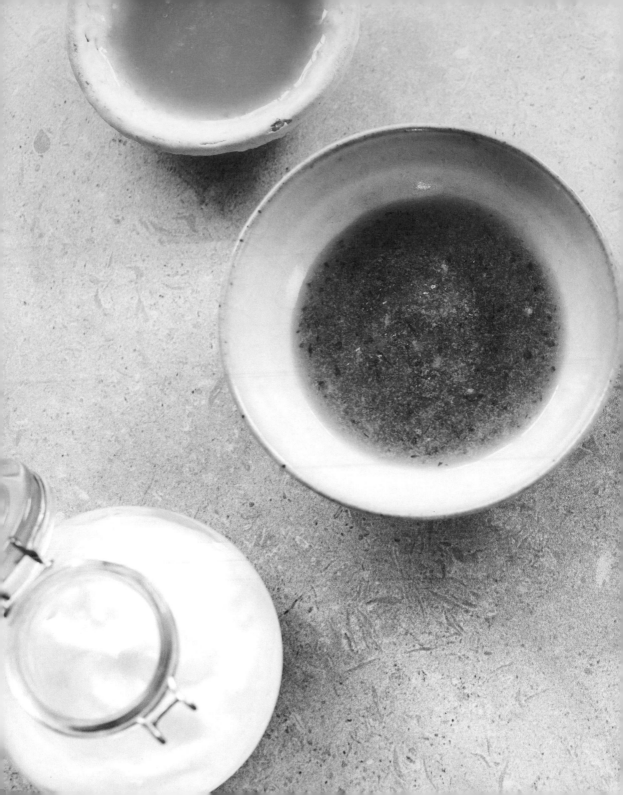

eye treatments

Taking care of the delicate skin around our eyes is essential for a more youthful appearance. The skin around the eyes is different to the rest of the skin on our bodies as it is much thinner, so it's one of the first areas to show signs of aging. Thinner skin means less fat cells and it will lose it's elasticity faster, resulting in a sunken look under the eyes and more lines. When we get sick, it's our eyes and the area around them that easily shows we are not well. So it's very important to make sure we keep ourselves well hydrated, have plenty of sleep and keep ourselves healthy and feeling good.

It's also super important to use eye creams that are specifically for the skin around the eyes, and ones that contain an SPF factor. It's not advised to use a regular skin cream as it will be too heavy for the thinner skin surrounding the eye.

In this chapter, I've included a few homemade treatments that I use regularly for calming and soothing tired eyes, decreasing puffiness, and some natural moisturizers to keep the skin hydrated. All the ingredients are natural and have vitamins and minerals that will gently nourish and rejuvenate the delicate eye area.

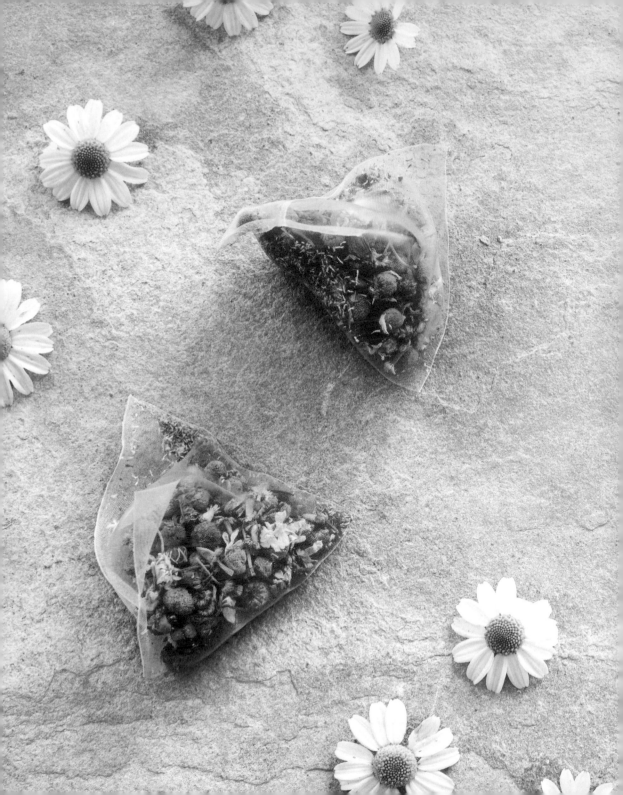

Chamomile Tea Soother

for tired, puffy eyes

The chamomile flower has been used for thousands of years in natural remedies. It contains significant anti-inflammatory and antimicrobial properties. When used directly on the skin of the eye area, it can help to reduce puffiness and soothe sore, tired skin.

2 chamomile teabags
hot water

Makes 1 application
Use immediately

This is really easy – simply put both of the teabags into a cup or mug and pour in just enough hot water to cover them. Let them steep for 10 seconds, then take them out and leave them to cool down to room temperature.

Remove all traces of make-up from your eyes. Lie back, close your eyes and place a teabag over each eye. Relax for 15 minutes, then remove the teabags and gently wash and dry your eye area.

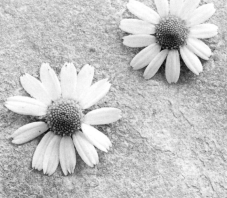

Cucumber + Aloe Vera Eye Gel

for sore, puffy and tired eyes

Cucumbers are a natural ingredient that are commonly used for their gentle and calming effects on the delicate skin around the eyes. This is because cucumbers are rich in antioxidants and flavonoids, which help to reduce redness, swelling and irritation. Aloe vera gel contains a phenomenal amount of vitamins, minerals and nutrients to help heal and soothe. A combination of the two makes a beautifully balanced natural eye remedy.

2.5-cm/1-inch piece of fresh cucumber
2 teaspoons pure aloe vera gel

Makes 1–2 applications
Keeps for up to 2 days in the refrigerator

Put the cucumber and aloe vera gel in a small food processor and blend to a fine purée, or use a pestle and mortar.

Remove all traces of make-up from your eyes. Gently apply the purée to the area underneath your eyes, around the outer corners and just under the brow bone, using either your fingertips or a small face-mask brush. You can also apply some to two cotton wool pads and place them over your closed eyes. Leave for 15 minutes, then gently wash off with warm water and pat dry.

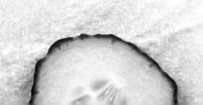

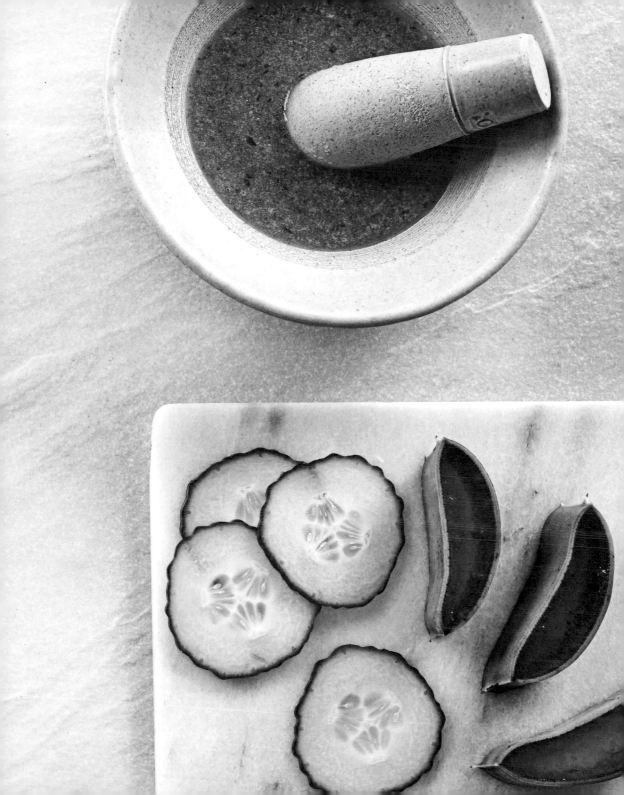

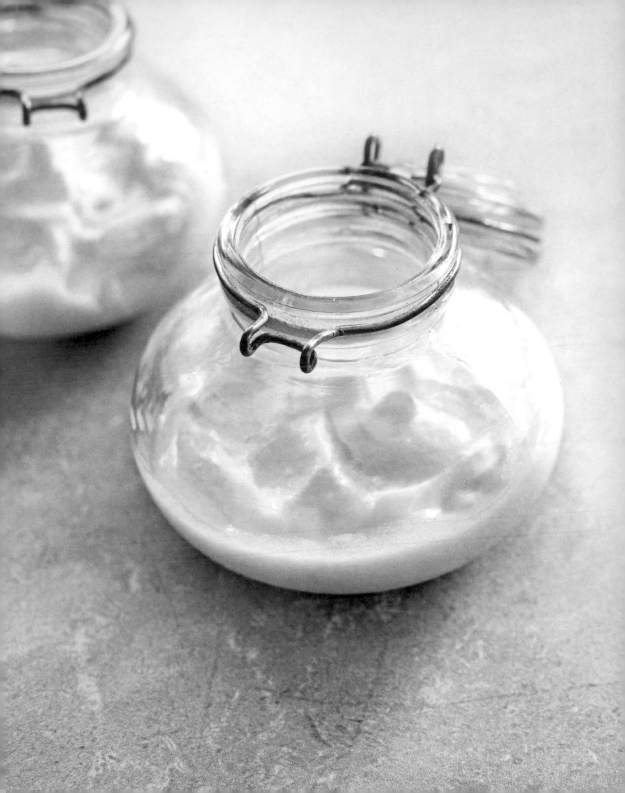

Night Eye Cream

all skin types

This luxurious eye cream is a great way to fight fine lines and keep the delicate skin around the eyes looking at its best. Cocoa butter is derived from the cocoa bean and is full of natural antioxidants. With its rich moisturizing properties, it helps the skin around the eyes maintain its elasticity. It is easily absorbed into the skin, so you don't have to rub or tug the skin when applying it, simply dab a little on the area underneath the eyes and let it soak in while you sleep.

20 g/¾ oz grated raw cocoa butter
2 tablespoons pure organic
*   coconut oil*
2 tablespoons pure aloe vera gel
1 teaspoon pure vitamin E oil

Makes approximately 60 g/2¼ oz/¼ cup

Keeps for up to 1 month if stored in an airtight jar, out of direct sunlight, ideally in your bathroom cupboard

Gently melt the cocoa butter and coconut oil together in a double boiler (a small heatproof bowl set over a saucepan of simmering water), or in a microwave on its lowest setting for a few seconds. Remove from the heat, leave to cool for a few minutes, then place the bowl in the freezer for 10 minutes. Once you see it beginning to solidify around the sides, take it out and add the rest of the ingredients. Using an electric whisk, beat until fluffy. If it is still runny and not turning fluffy, put it back in the freezer for another couple of minutes, then take it out and beat again for a few seconds. The consistency should be a light, soft cream.

Remove all traces of make-up from your eyes. Using your fingertips, gently dab a small amount of the cream onto the area underneath your eyes, around the outer corners and just under the brow bone. Let the cream absorb into the skin. This is best applied before going to bed at night.

Note: You can substitute the coconut oil for almond oil or jojoba oil, if you prefer.

Coffee Under-eye Mask

tired and puffy eyes

Coffee is widely used in beauty regimes as the caffeine has a tightening effect on the skin and helps to reduce puffiness and dark circles under the eyes. The coffee berry powder adds powerful antioxidants that help to fight free radicals that can damage skin cells. Aloe vera gel is gentle, soothing and nourishing for the delicate skin, and the vitamin E oil is moisturizing.

1 tablespoon ground coffee
½ teaspoon coffee berry powder
1 tablespoon pure aloe vera gel
2 drops pure vitamin E oil

Makes 2 applications
Keeps for up to 2–3 days in the refrigerator

Put all the ingredients in a small bowl and mix together.

Remove all traces of make-up from your eyes. Using a small face-mask brush or your fingertips, gently apply a thick layer of the eye mask to the area underneath the eyes. Lie down and relax for 10 minutes, then gently wash it off with warm water and pat dry.

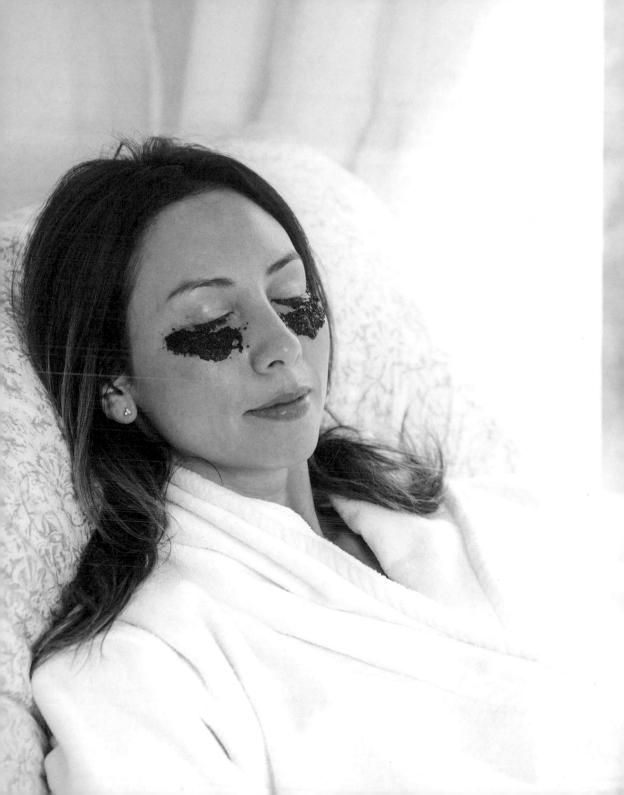

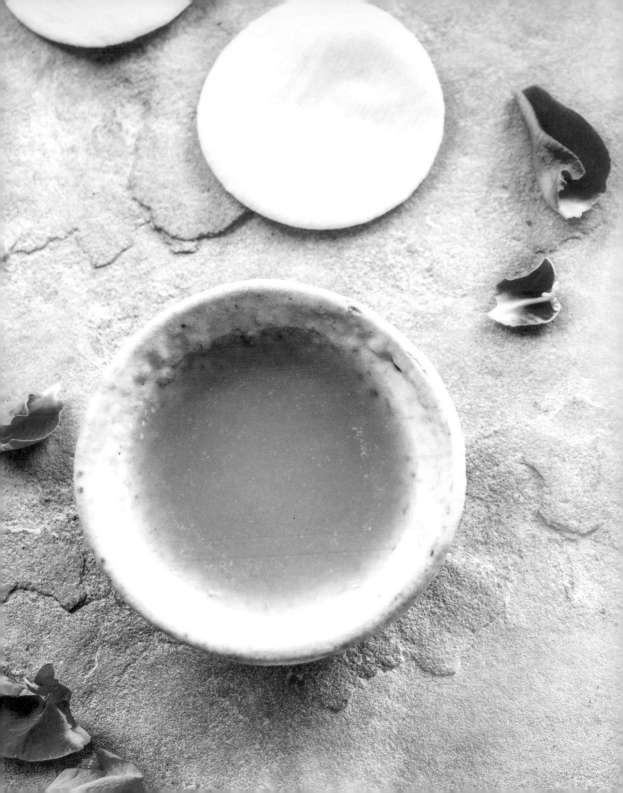

Rosewater + Potato Juice Cooling Eye Pads

all skin types

Potatoes contain an astringent that helps to remove excess water from the skin, which is why it is popular to place a slice of potato under the eyes to reduce puffiness. I love using rosewater as it's so gentle and smells gorgeous, so I mixed these two wonderful ingredients together to make soothing eye pads. Rosewater is also a natural astringent, so you're getting a double dose of puffiness reduction, plus it helps to rejuvenate tired eyes.

½ medium-sized potato
1 tablespoon pure rosewater

Makes enough for 2–3 applications
Keeps for only a day in the refrigerator, so this is a good one to share

Peel the potato and grate it into a bowl. Using your hands, squeeze a small handful of the grated potato so that all the juice comes out. Place the squeezed potato into another bowl; it's the juice you want to keep. Continue squeezing until you've squeezed all the potato. It won't make much juice, perhaps a couple of tablespoonfuls, but that's all you need. Add the rosewater to the potato juice and mix together. Pour the solution into a clean container with a lid and leave it to chill in the refrigerator for at least 2 hours. You want it to be nice and cold when you apply it, as the cool temperature also helps to reduce puffiness.

When it's cold enough, take two cotton wool pads or eye sponges and soak them in the mixture. Remove all traces of eye make-up, then sit back, close your eyes, place the pads or sponges on top and relax for 15 minutes. Remove the eye pads or sponges and gently wash the area around the eyes with cold water. Pat the skin dry, then moisturize with your favourite eye cream.

Note: You can use the grated potato to make potato cakes or traditional Jewish latkes.

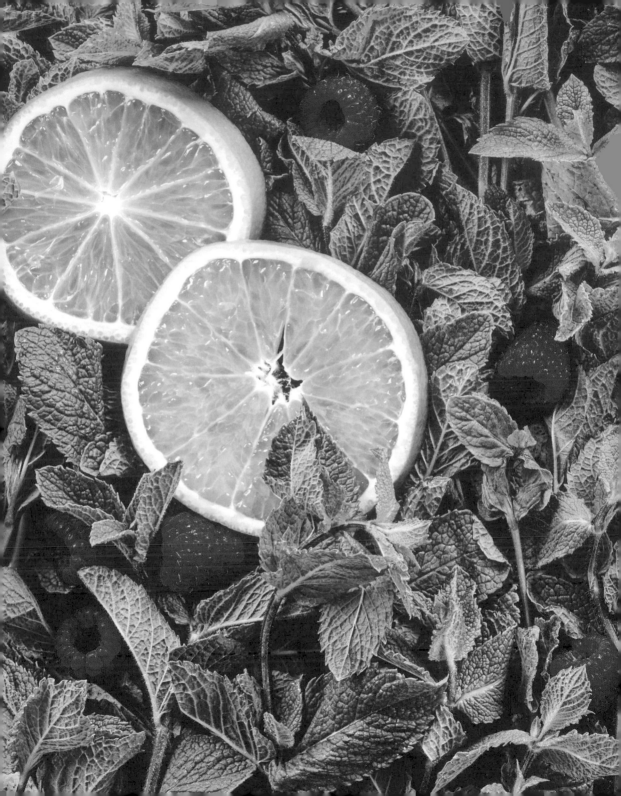

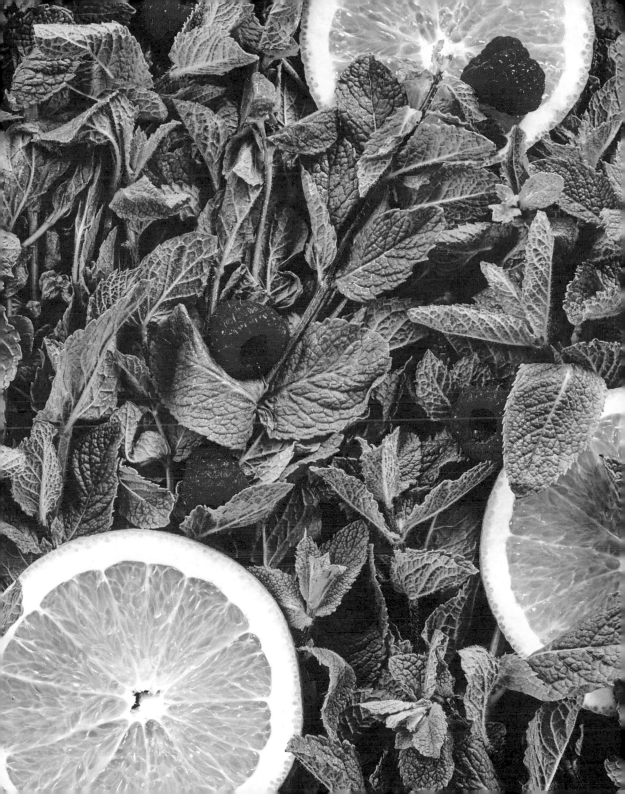

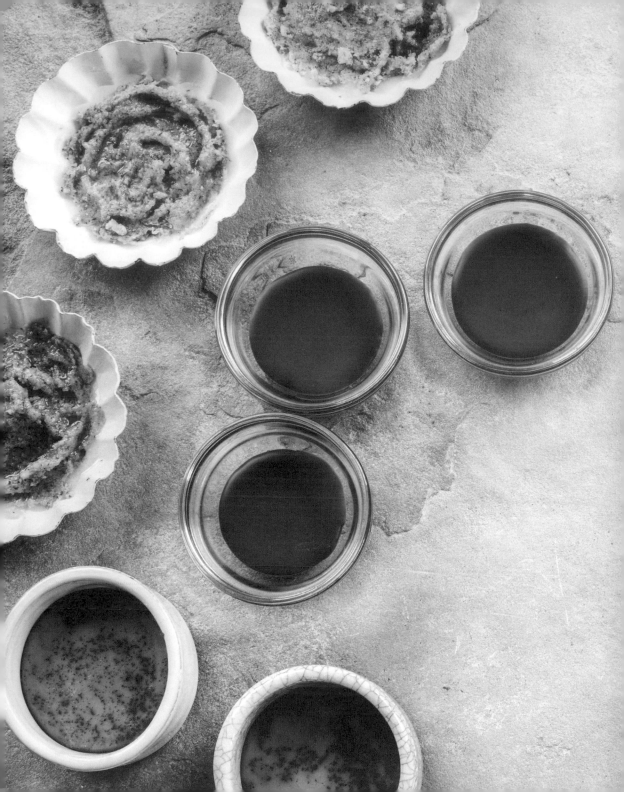

lip remedies

I've always been a real sucker for lip products, I adore them, and I love having soft, moisturized lips. One way to keep lips soft and supple is to do a weekly exfoliation. The great thing is you can make your own gorgeous sugar lip scrubs at home to keep chapped lips at bay.

Exfoliating dry chapped lips helps get rid of the dead skin, and then when you moisturize using a lip balm, the ingredients get absorbed properly into your skin. The skin on your lips is very delicate, so you only need to do the scrub once or twice a week. I just use my finger to rub the scrub in gently, then use a facecloth to wipe it off.

I've included my favourite scrubs and moisturizing recipes for your lips, but once you know the basics, you can experiment and make your own favourite flavours. I've had great fun turning my kitchen into an apothecary and experimenting with different flavours, colours and aromas.

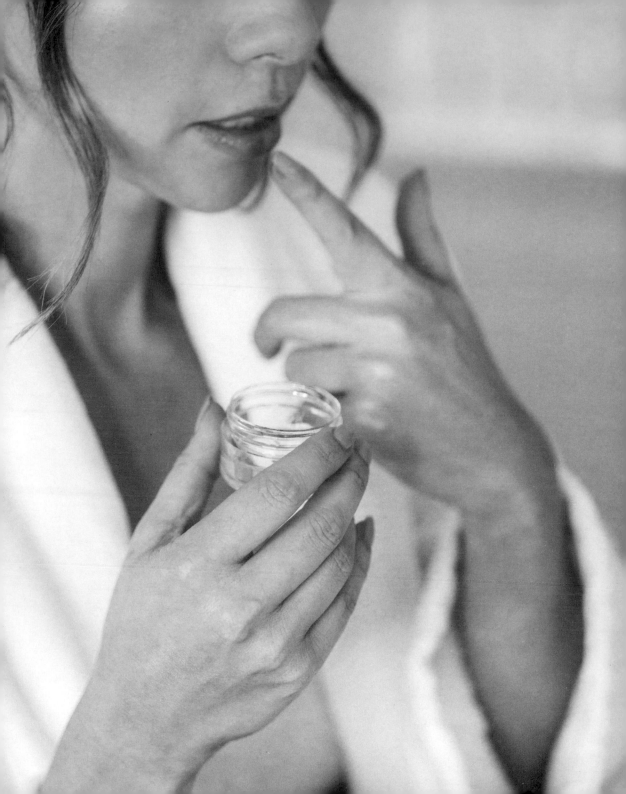

Vitamin E + Avocado Oil Lip Moisturizer
dry chapped lips

Vitamin E is a powerful antioxidant that can help to prevent sun damage and dry, chapped lips. I tend to put sunscreen on all over and then forget about my lips, so I keep this soothing oil in a pot to put on my lips before I go to bed. Avocado oil is packed full of good fats and vitamin E to help keep the lips soft. Lemon essential oil has antibacterial properties to ward off any infections, and I love the smell of sweet orange essential oil, so I add a couple of drops of that, too.

1 teaspoon pure vitamin E oil
1 tablespoon pure avocado oil
1 drop lemon essential oil
2 drops sweet orange essential oil

Makes 30 applications

Keeps for up to 4–6 weeks in a small (45-ml/1½-oz) jar with a lid

Put all the ingredients in a small bowl and mix together. Pour the oil into a small, clean storage jar with a lid.

Using a cotton bud/Q-tip or fingertip, dab a little on your lips before bedtime. A little goes a long way.

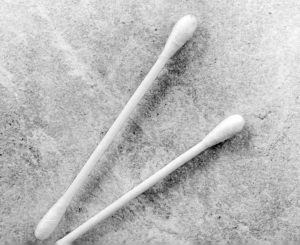

Peppermint Sugar + Shea Butter Lip Scrub

all lips

The peppermint essential oil combined with the fresh mint and raw shea butter make an invigorating and gentle lip scrub that will leave your lips minty fresh and soft.

2 teaspoons pure raw shea butter
4 fresh mint leaves (optional)
1 tablespoon white granulated sugar
5 drops peppermint essential oil

Makes 15–20 applications
Keeps for up to 1 month in a small (45-ml/1½-oz) jar with a lid

Gently melt the shea butter in a double boiler (a small heatproof bowl set over a saucepan of simmering water), or in a microwave on its lowest setting for a few seconds. Leave to cool slightly. If using fresh mint leaves, put them in a small food processor with the sugar and whizz until the mint leaves are finely chopped. Put the mint and sugar into a small bowl, add the peppermint essential oil and melted shea butter and mix together to form a paste. Spoon into a small jar with a lid.

When your lips feel dry and cracked, take a little of the scrub, about ½ teaspoonful, and massage it gently into your lips with your fingertip for about a minute. Wipe it off with a warm, damp facecloth or just wash it off with water, and pat your lips dry.

Honey + Lemon Chapped Lips Sugar Scrub

dry chapped lips

This is a super-easy remedy to make at home with easily available ingredients. Raw honey has many healing properties and is even used on open wounds to help them heal quicker.

½ teaspoon organic raw honey
1 teaspoon freshly squeezed lemon juice
1 drop lemon essential oil (optional)

4 teaspoons white granulated sugar

Makes 20 applications
Keeps for up to 2 weeks in a small (45-ml/1½-oz) jar with a lid

Put all the ingredients in a small bowl and mix together to create a thick scrub. Use the scrub whenever your lips are feeling dry. Simply massage a little onto your lips with your fingertip for about a minute, then wipe it off with a warm, damp facecloth or just wash it off with water.

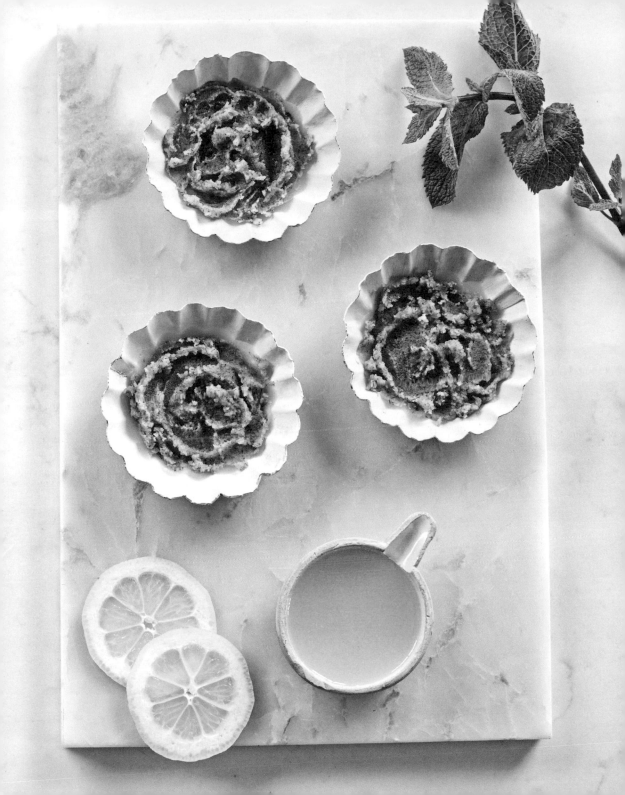

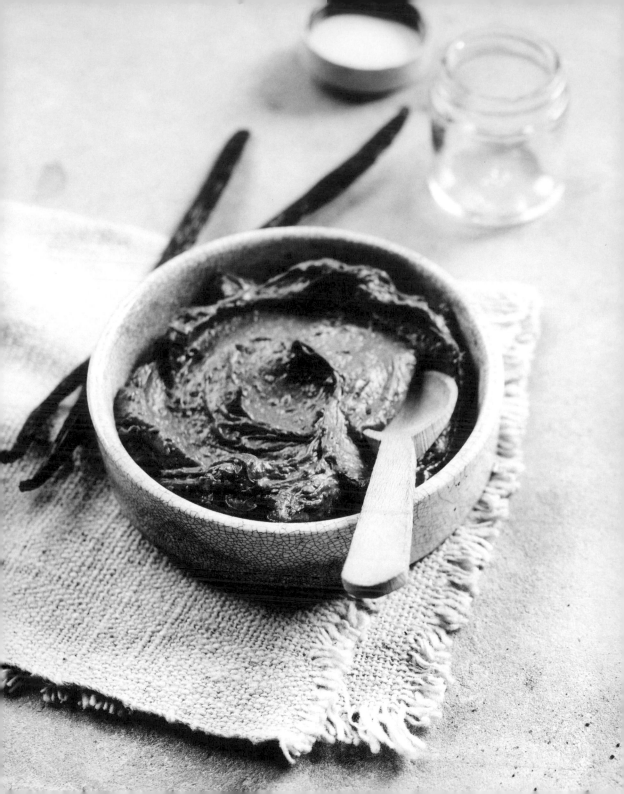

Cocoa Butter Lips

all lips

Cocoa butter is a divine-smelling, healthy, skin-friendly fat derived from the cocoa bean that makes chocolate. Yes, that's right, this lip balm will smell and taste like chocolate, so you might have a hard time trying not to lick your lips. Cocoa butter contains emollients that leave a protective and moisturizing layer on your lips.

1½ tablespoons grated raw cocoa butter
1½ teaspoons pure organic coconut oil or pure jojoba oil
1 teaspoon pure unsweetened cocoa powder
½ teaspoon pure vanilla extract
10 drops pure vitamin E oil

Makes approx. 50 applications
Keeps for up to a month in a small (45ml/1½oz) jar with a lid

Gently melt the cocoa butter and coconut oil together in a double boiler (a small heatproof bowl set over a saucepan of simmering water), or in a microwave on its lowest setting for a few seconds. Remove from the heat, leave to cool for a few minutes, then place the bowl in the freezer for 10 minutes. Once you see it beginning to solidify around the sides, take it out and add the rest of the ingredients. Using an electric whisk, beat until fluffy. If it is still runny and not turning fluffy, put it back in the freezer for another couple of minutes as it needs to cool down to the right temperature to set. Take it out and beat again for a few seconds until it turns fluffy and holds it shape. Transfer to a small jar with a lid.

Use this delicious lip balm whenever your lips feel dry, simply patting a little over your lips with your fingertip.

Raspberry Lip Balm

all lips

Once you have all the right ingredients it's very easy to make your own lip balm – and once you start, you'll never go back to the store-bought variety. Beeswax is the key ingredient here; it's completely natural, it makes the lip balm stay hard, plus it's an excellent lip protector and moisturizer. I have added in some extra moisturizing ingredients, in the form of vitamin E oil and jojoba oil, to take good care of your luscious lips. The raspberries give your lips a slight hint of pink the natural way.

1½ tablespoons freeze-dried raspberries
2 tablespoons pure jojoba oil
1½ teaspoons natural beeswax pellets (see note)
10 drops pure vitamin E oil
1 drop rose or lavender essential oil (optional)

Makes approx. 50 applications
Keeps for up to a month in a small (45 ml/1½ oz) jar with a lid

Grind the freeze-dried raspberries in a coffee grinder or small food processor until very fine. Gently heat the jojoba oil and beeswax together in a double boiler (a small heatproof bowl set over a saucepan of simmering water), or in a microwave on its lowest setting for a few seconds. When melted, remove from the heat and add the vitamin E oil, raspberry powder and, if you wish, a drop of rose or lavender essential oil. Pour the mixture into a little jar with a lid, and leave to set.

The raspberry powder can feel a bit grainy on the lips, but I rub my lips together and use it like an exfoliant, too, leaving my lips feeling super-soft.

Note: I find it easier to buy beeswax in pellet form, as the blocks are difficult to cut for small quantities.

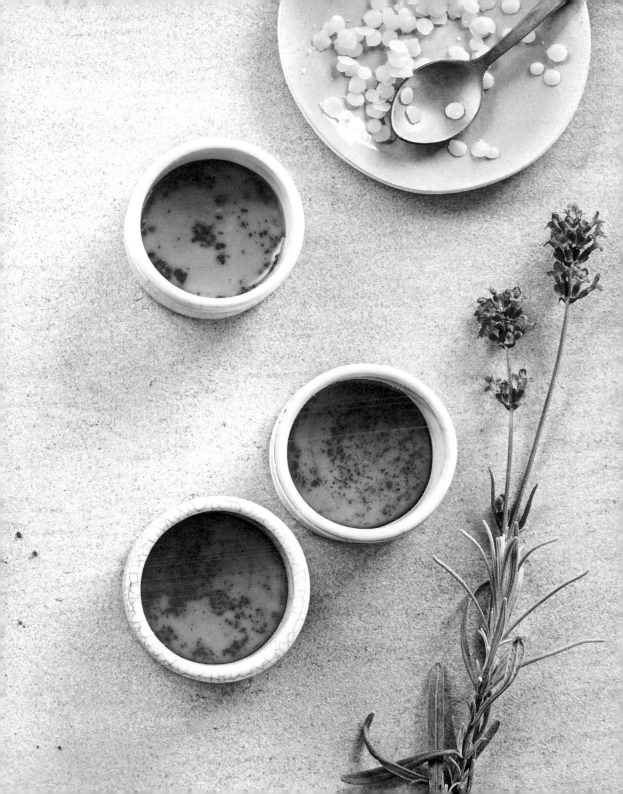

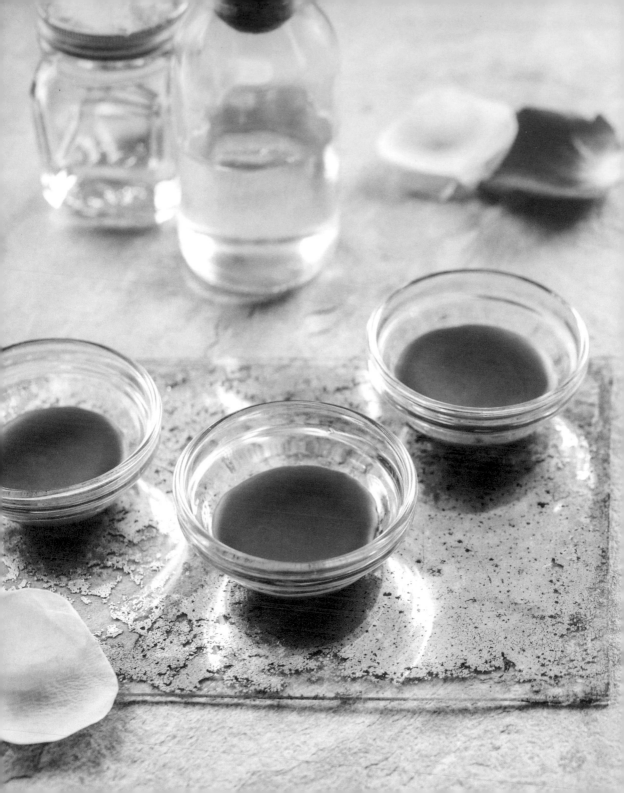

Tinted Rose Lip Balm

all lips

Beeswax is a natural lip and skin defender as it leaves a layer on the surface, locking moisture in and forming a protective barrier against air and other elements. Vitamin E is an antioxidant that helps protect the skin cells from sun damage and can also speed up the natural healing process, so it works wonders on dry, cracked lips. This lip balm has a hint of colour, which can be provided by old lipsticks that you can use up or, if you prefer, a completely natural dye – you can find ones online made from food sources such as beetroot or paprika.

2 tablespoons pure jojoba oil
1½ teaspoons natural beeswax pellets
¼ of a coloured lipstick of your choice, or a few drops of natural dye
10 drops pure vitamin E oil
3 drops rose essential oil (optional)

Makes approx. 50 applications
Keeps for 4–6 weeks in a small (45-ml/1½ oz) jar with a lid

Gently heat the jojoba oil, beeswax and piece of lipstick or natural dye together in a double boiler (a small heatproof bowl set over a saucepan of simmering water), or in a microwave on its lowest setting for a few seconds. Stir the mixture so the lipstick melts down, then remove from the heat and add the vitamin E oil and rose essential oil. Pour the mixture into a little jar with a lid and leave it to set.

Apply the lip balm to your lips with your fingertip or a lip brush.

Note: If you want to make a lip balm with a stronger colour, just add a larger piece of lipstick or more dye. If you don't want any colour, leave this ingredient out.

Index

Acknowledgments

First, I'd like to say how grateful I am to have been asked by Ryland Peters & Small Publishers to write my second book with them. It's a true pleasure to be given the opportunity to create the recipes and have them published in this beautifully presented book. Thank you to the talented team of editors, designers, photographers and food stylists who helped bring this book to life and to my book agent Alan Nevins at Renaissance Literary and Talent, Los Angeles.

I wouldn't have been able to achieve all I have without the momentous support of my family. My sisters Rose and Michelle for taste-testing all my strange concoctions growing up. My little brother Alex, who will always be my dear baby brother no matter how old you are. My late father, David, for teaching me his love of food. My step-father, Michael, for the constant support, plus the many taxi service lifts you have provided me over the years to and fro the airport. My beautiful daughter, Bethany, for modelling in this book, for being my greatest teacher in life, my toughest critic and the most wonderful thing to ever happen to me.

To my late mother, whose tremendous knowledge and years of experience in the beauty clinic world inspired me to write the recipes in this book. Not only were her words of wisdom invaluable to my own beauty regime, I'm so happy they will also be passed on to everyone who reads this book, so they too can enjoy healthy, clear and beautiful skin.

To all my close friends, you know who you are, my life wouldn't be as bright without you. Thank you for being my guinea pigs.

Lastly, to you reading this book, a huge heart-felt thank you. I truly hope you enjoy using my beauty masks and that you find your favourite natural treatments to help you glow a bit brighter than you already are.

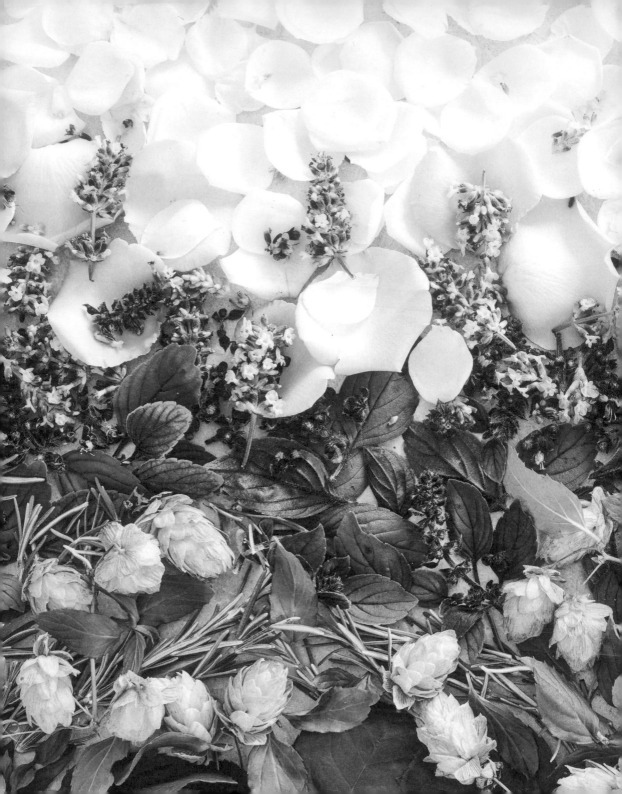